The Essentials of
Paediatrics for Nurses

The Essentials of Paediatrics for Nurses

I. KESSEL
M.B., B.Ch., F.R.C.P.(Lond.), F.R.C.P.(Edin.), D.C.H.(Eng.)

Consultant Paediatrician, North West Thames Regional Health
Authority (Watford General Hospital, Hemel Hempstead General
Hospital and Leavesden Hospital).
Honorary Associate Physician, Hospital for Sick Children,
Great Ormond Street, London.
Formerly Senior Paediatrician, Transvaal Memorial Hospital
for Children and the University of the Witwatersrand,
Johannesburg, South Africa

FIFTH EDITION

CHURCHILL LIVINGSTONE
Edinburgh London and New York 1976

CHURCHILL LIVINGSTONE
Medical Division of Longman Group Limited

Distributed in the United States of America by
Longman Inc., 19 West 44th Street, New York,
N.Y. 10036 and by associated companies,
branches and representatives throughout the world.

First Edition 1957
Second Edition 1963
Third Edition 1967
Fourth Edition 1972
Fifth Edition 1976
Reprinted   1977

ISBN 0 443 01420 5

Library of Congress Cataloging in Publication Data

Kessel, Israel.
  The essentials of paediatrics for nurses.

  Includes index.
  1. Pediatrics. 2. Pediatric nursing. I. Title.
(DNLM: 1. Pediatric nursing. WY159 K42e)
RJ45.K44 1976   618.9′2   75-43553

Printed in Hong Kong by Commonwealth Printing Press Ltd

This book is dedicated to
my late dear wife
Elizabeth Hannah Kessel, S.R.N., S.C.M.

Preface to the Fifth Edition

THERE have been a number of new developments in the application of knowledge in paediatrics and also in medicine generally and this has led to the need for having a fifth edition of this book within a relatively short space of time since the appearance of the fourth edition. The importance of the neonatal period has remained and has even become more so in recent years and has had added to this the strides that have been made into the prenatal period. Various sections have been rewritten in relation to these advances and some new sections have been added and also some new poisons have been described. New illustrations have been included in an attempt to enhance the educational value of this book.

I must acknowledge the great assistance given to me by Margaret Wood in the important secretarial duties associated with the compilation of this edition and her patience and efficiency was especially noteworthy. My late dear wife Elizabeth continually helped me in revising and reading the manuscripts of the previous editions and without her support and assistance these editions could not have been prepared. My daughter, Patricia, and son, Jonathan, have continued to help me with the new manuscript. I again express my gratitude to my colleagues who provided me with the clinical material for the illustrations included from the first four editions; my thanks also go to Vickers Limited and KeyMed Specialised Medical Equipment Limited. I am extremely grateful to Dr B. Cheng, Consultant Chemical Pathologist to the Watford General Hospital, for his list and comments on the normal ranges of laboratory investigations in biochemistry in the new SI system. I must also acknowledge my deep appreciation to the nursing staff of the paediatric, obstetric and teaching departments and the special care baby units of the Watford General Hospital and the Hemel Hempstead General Hospital for their efforts in allowing me to appreciate recent trends of thought in the nursing field. My continuing discussions with the nursing staff of the children's wards including Sisters D. V. Nash, I. A. Bentley and L. Boyes and Miss J. E. Wilkinson have been of considerable assistance to me.

Finally I must express my gratitude to my publishers, Churchill Livingstone, for their guidance and support and patience in producing this new edition.

I. KESSEL

London, 1976

Preface to the First Edition

THIS book has been written to meet most of the medical require-ments for paediatric nurses. Stress has been laid throughout the book on the basic principles of this important branch of Medicine, especially in relation to modern trends and advances in this subject. Many standard textbooks on Paediatrics and Child Health have been constantly referred to and also numerous journals dealing with the health of infants and children; they are too numerous to mention singly but I would wish a general acknowledgement to be made and express my sincere thanks to these publications. I would like to stress that this book does not attempt to discuss nursing procedures in relation to the sick child; there are many excellent publications available which cover this field.

My thanks are due to Miss M. L. A. Hills whose time-consuming task in typing the manuscript was worthy of the highest praise. My wife assisted me throughout the writing and reading of the manuscript. I must express my thanks to Dr K. F. Mills, Medical Superintendent, Johannesburg Hospital, for his permission to use illustrations of material in the Hospital, to Dr Seymour Heymann, Head of the Depart-ment of Paediatrics, University of the Witwatersrand and the Transvaal Memorial Hospital for Children, for allowing me to use his clinical cases for illustrations, and to Prof. O. S. Heyns, Professor of Obstetrics and Gynaecology, University of the Witwatersrand, Dr L. G. R. Van Dongen and Dr F. Daubenton of the same Department, for making available to me their clinical cases of neonatal conditions; detailed acknowledgement for the use of other clinical material for illustrations and for other matter is made separately. I would like to express my gratitude to Dr S. Wayburne, Paediatrician, Baragwanath Hospital, for his kindness in allowing me to use his photographs of nutritional cases and others, chosen from his excellent collection of photographic material—the finest I have seen. I must also acknowledge gratefully the assistance given me in the clinical photography by Mr A. M. Shevitz (Department of Medicine, University of the Witwatersrand), Dr H. Sher and Mr J. I. Van Niekerk (Department of Obstetrics and Gynae-cology, University of the Witwatersrand). I must also thank Sisters I. McLellan and A. M. Mackay for their kind assistance and Staff Nurse P. M. Lacey for her help with the tables.

Finally, I must express my gratitude to Mr Charles Macmillan of E. & S. Livingstone for his lasting patience with me.

Johannesburg,
November, 1956   I. KESSEL

Acknowledgements

The sincere thanks of the author are due to the following for the use of their clinical material from which illustrations were made, for illustrations and for other matter used in this book:

Dr J. Adno, Miss S. M. Bekhit, Dr B. Cheng, Yvonne Cowey, Dr M. Culloty, Prof. F. Daubenton, Prof. L. G. R. van Dongen, Prof. A. E. H. Emery, Dr F. C. Friedlander, Prof. H. Glietenberg, Dr Z. Harary, Dr Seymour C. Heymann, Dr S. N. Javett, Dr P. Kushlick, Mr J. Lannon, Dr G. Marks, Dr M. Medalie, Dr I. Nessim, Dr J. L. Parnell, Prof. G. H. Percival, Prof. N. S. F. Proctor, Dr J. M. Samson, Dr R. J. S. Sichel, Mr J. N. Smith, Miss M. J. Symonds, Dr J. J. Theron, Dr H. L. Utian, Sister E. A. Vincent, Prof. D. H. Walker, Prof. S. Wayburne, Dr C. Glynn Williams, Dr Victor Berman and the Department of Radiology, Transvaal Memorial Hospital for Children, The General Nursing Council for England and Wales, The South African Nursing Council, The Editor of *Archives of Disease in Childhood*, The Editor of *British Medical Journal*, The Editor of *Journal of Obstetrics and Gynaecology of the British Commonwealth*, The Editor of *The Journal of Pediatrics*, The Editor of *South African Practitioner*, Vickers Limited, KeyMed Specialised Medical Equipment Limited.

Contents

1. The Normal Child and Developmental Paediatrics

The development of an individual is a continuous process and must be seen as starting at conception and continuing to maturity. This continuous developmental process is controlled by the maturing nervous system.

The normal is usually very difficult to define and there is a wide range of normality in most things; this applies very much to medicine generally and also to the assessment of the normal infant and child. There are a number of primitive reflexes present in the normal newborn infant such as the grasp reflex.

In an infant and child this normal development, both physical and mental, has this wide range and it is necessary that those who deal with the care of the infant and child should have a basic approach and knowledge of average development in order to assess properly the patients under their care. Comprehensive assessment centres are essential for the management of the handicapped child and these centres are necessary in maintaining proper child health services. From the practical point of view in order to assess physical growth in infancy and childhood it is necessary to use certain measurements and the most appropriate of these indices of measurement are those of length (or height) and weight. It is essential to have accuracy in taking these measurements and proper techniques for the measurement of supine length and stature are required. Weight is an easier measurement but is not as useful for growth studies of the individual. Charts of height and weight and their velocities are available in which the usual standards are given as centiles. If a child is at the third centile then 3 per cent of children are less tall or growing less fast. If at the fiftieth centile then 50 per cent of children are smaller and if at the ninety-seventh centile, 97 per cent are smaller. There are various other features of importance in the physical development of a child and, in addition, mental developmental milestones are important in assessing the normal infant.

Weight

In the last trimester of pregnancy there is a rapid rate of growth in the foetus. After birth there is an early rapid increase followed by a slower phase of growth until puberty when there is again a rapid

1

advance with the adolescent spurt of growth, although in a few children there appears to be a slight increase in velocity between 6 and 8 years. At birth the average weight is approximately 3500 g, there is a small drop in the first few days and the birth weight is regained by approximately the tenth day. A steady gain then occurs so that the birth weight is doubled by the fifth month and trebled by the end of the first year. This is followed by a slower increase so that the following approximate weights are attained: 13 kg at 2 years; 15 kg at 3 years; 25 kg at 8 years; and 30 kg at 10 years.

There has been a general tendency for the weight and height standards of normal children to be higher than those of many decades ago and this tendency is still slowly continuing.

Length (or Height)

At birth the normal length is 50 cm. In the premature infant it has been said that double the length expressed in inches is approximately equal to the period of gestation expressed in weeks although there are more satisfactory methods available to determine the period of gestation more accurately. The length at birth is approximately doubled at 4 years and from about 6 years about 5 cm per year are added in height until approximately the eleventh year. About 22·5 cm are added in the first year of life and approximately 10 cm in the second and third years. After the age of about 4 or 5 years, a child takes on some of the hereditary growth characteristics of its parents and it is essential to allow for this parental height.

The skull

At birth the circumference of the skull is about 35 cm. This increases rapidly in the first year so that the circumference reaches about 42 cm at 6 months and about 47 cm at a year. After this, the skull grows at a slower rate; the circumference at 3 years is about 50 cm and at 8 years approximately 53 cm. This increase in size of the skull is representative of the increasing growth of the brain. At birth there are six fontanelles present, the one of principal importance being the anterior fontanelle, which is situated at the anterior end of the sagittal suture where it meets with the coronal sutures. This anterior fontanelle slowly diminishes in size until it is completely closed by about the eighteenth month after birth; it may remain open longer in such conditions as hydrocephalus, rickets and cretinism. There is a wide range of normal in the size of the anterior fontanelle and in normal infants it may be small and close early. The posterior, or occipital, fontanelle, which is situated at the posterior end of the sagittal suture where it joins with the lambdoid suture, is closed at birth in a fair proportion of infants; in the remainder, it closes by the third month.

The teeth

The deciduous or milk teeth start erupting at about the sixth month; the first to appear are the lower central incisors, followed by the upper. At about 9 months, the lateral incisors erupt and are followed by the first molars at a variable time from the fifteenth to the eighteenth month. The canines then appear at about 18 months, and finally, at about 2 years, the second molars erupt to complete the 20 teeth of the deciduous dentition. As a rule the lower teeth, except for the lateral incisors, erupt before their counterparts in the upper jaw. The permanent teeth start erupting at the age of 6 years with the appearance of the first molars. The permanent dentition is completed by the eruption of the second molars at about 12 years of age, except for the wisdom teeth or third molars, which appear much later, near the age of 18 to 20 years.

Miscellaneous physical features

The pulse rate at birth is about 130 per minute. This gradually becomes slower, being about 100 per minute at 2 years, 95 at 3 years and 90 at 7 years. The systolic blood pressure gradually rises from birth onwards. A newborn infant can distinguish heat from cold and light from darkness. At about 4 weeks of age a bright light may be followed and at 4 months the child can observe detail. Loud noises may be heard in the second week and from then onwards hearing improves steadily. The newborn infant has well developed senses of smell and taste. The very young infant sleeps almost the whole 24 hours; this sleep period gradually lessens so that by a year about 15 hours are spent in sleep, and 12 hours at 3 years.

Milestones of development (mental development)

A normal infant can hold up his head at about 3 to 4 months and can sit up unsupported from 6 to 9 months. There are more detailed methods of assessing development and these include the handling of toys: at 2 months a rattle will be followed by the eyes briefly and a month later it will be held in the hand when placed there; at 4 months toys will be put in the mouth and at 5 to 6 months a normal infant will reach out and grasp a toy with one hand; a toy may be handled in each hand at 8 months and a month later will be grasped with the thumb and index finger. Between the ages of 12 and 18 months most infants stand unaided and can walk a few steps, but even normal children may be delayed in this. Talking starts at a variable age: some infants use simple single words at 1 year whereas others do not start until the age of 2 years. Failure to talk by 2 years may be regarded as backwardness in speech; the cause, however, may not be mental retardation but may be associated with deafness. Many developmental tests in the infant and young child have been devised but there has been controversy as to their value in predicting future development. Developmental tests of infants are of value and are essential in assessing possible cases of mental retardation and neurological abnormality. It is necessary to stress also that deafness should be detected as early as possible, preferably in the first year; specially trained observers are available to undertake routine hearing tests in the first year. If detected, auditory training can commence as early as possible and hearing aids are being used successfully in young infants.

Vision defects may be caused by detectable cataracts and also squints which are both treatable. Vision testing in early life is available using STYCAR methods (screening tests for young children and retardates) and other tests.

Developmental paediatrics

The development of comprehensive assessment centres for handicapped children are essential in maintaining a proper overall child health service. It is recognised that the care and assessment of the normal and the handicapped child is no less important than the management of the sick child and developmental paediatrics is an important necessary field in a child health service.

Improving child health services have led to a decline in infant mortality and morbidity and this in turn has led to the increasing survival of children with physical and mental defects with, in many cases, their accompanying emotional problems.

Comprehensive assessment centres for the handicapped child require a service to help in developing the best available talents in such a child to the greatest ability. Some of the conditions associated with the handicapped child may be diagnosed at birth (for example, Down's syndrome (mongolism) and multiple congenital deformities); other conditions may be suspected by routine screening procedures (for example, congenital dislocation of the hip, deafness, vision defects and phenylketonuria); other conditions may only become apparent later (for example, cerebral palsy and mental subnormality).

2. Low Birth Weight

Very great importance is being placed on low birth weight and this includes the low birth weight for gestation ('small-for-dates' or 'light-for-dates') infant. The low birth weight infants can be divided into different categories as follows: (1) infants of low birth weight who are prematurely delivered before 37 weeks with a weight appropriate for the gestational age, (2) infants of low birth weight born after a normal gestational period but who are lighter than expected for the gestational age, (3) infants of low birth weight born prematurely and of a weight less than expected for the gestational age. The importance of these low birth weight infants is partly related to neonatal and infant mortality rates. By definition, the neonatal mortality rate is the number of deaths of infants in the first four weeks of life per 1000 live births, while the infant mortality rate is the number of deaths of infants in the first year of life per 1000 live births. The stillbirth rate, which is unrelated to this discussion, is defined as the number of stillbirths per 1000 total births. Another important term used is perinatal mortality, which includes neonatal deaths and stillbirths and is therefore related to both foetal and neonatal loss.

In many countries both infant and neonatal mortality rates have been greatly reduced. A high proportion of neonatal deaths are due to the death of the low birth weight infant, and it is clear that if the neonatal mortality rate is to be further reduced, more low birth weight infants must be saved. A more logical approach to this problem would be an attempt to reduce the number of low birth weight infants that are born, by allowing more pregnancies to go to term. Approximately 7 per cent of infants are born with a weight below 2500 g of which about two-thirds are between 2000 and 2500 g and it is those below this category that give rise to many problems.

Definition
By international agreement a premature or low birth weight infant was defined as an infant with a birth weight of 2500 g or less. This definition is not physiologically accurate for a premature infant as such an infant is one born after the twenty-eighth week of gestation but before a term of 37 weeks gestation has elapsed.

Aetiology
Unfortunately a high proportion of low birth weight infants, up to about 50 per cent, occur without known cause. Of the known causes,

many are due to the toxaemias of pregnancy or to multiple pregnancy, such as twins; these constitute a high proportion of known causes. Other possible causes are related to placenta praevia and accidental haemorrhage and also acute illness in the mother, gross congenital abnormality of the infant and hydramnios may be associated with premature labour. The low birth weight for gestation ('small-for-dates') infant is associated with conditions which interfere with intrauterine growth and socioeconomic factors may be important and also maternal toxaemia and inadequate antenatal care. Another well recognised cause is smoking during pregnancy.

Clinical features

These features vary according to the size of the infant. By definition the weight at birth is 2500 g or less and the length is less than 50 cm. It has been said that the length of the preterm infant in inches is approximately half the period of gestation expressed in weeks, but other methods are used to assess gestational age apart from the calculation in relation to the mother's last menstrual period; this calculation may give rise to difficulty where the menstrual cycle is very irregular and also the widespread use of oral contraceptives ('The Pill') may confuse the dates. Ultrasonic scanning of the uterus and also amniotic fluid obtained by amniocentesis can be useful in obtaining information to assess the gestational age of the foetus by using such assessments as the difference in its urea content in comparison with that of the mother's blood urea level, the creatinine level of the fluid and also assessing the foetal skin cells. After birth a neurological assessment is very useful in assessing the gestational age. The appearance of certain neurological reflexes such as the glabella tap reflex which appears at 32 to 34 weeks gestation, the response of the pupils to light at 29 to 31 weeks, the neck retraction reflex at 34 to 37 weeks and the head turning to the light at 32 to 36 weeks. The Moro reflex is also useful but has a wide variation in relation to its appearing at certain gestational ages. The low birth weight infant has a weak vitality with poor respiratory function and a feeble cry. The pulse rate varies from 100 to 160 per minute with an average of 130. These infants have weak feeding ability and pass small amounts of urine. The skin is red and wrinkled and is covered with much lanugo hair. There is little subcutaneous fat present and the nails do not extend to the ends of the fingers. These infants cannot maintain their body temperatures and have but little resistance to infection.

Management

The management of the low birth weight infant may be discussed under certain headings:

1. Maintenance of body temperature
2. Establishment and maintenance of respiratory function

3. Prevention of infection
4. Feeding
5. Miscellaneous

Maintenance of body temperature. The low birth weight infant, especially the preterm, has not established the heat-regulating mechanism and so cannot maintain optimum body temperature. Heat is lost in many different ways, such as insensible loss, and also by convection and radiation. Heat loss by conduction is very small if the infant lies on a warm mattress with low conductivity. The radiant heat loss is important in the incubator care of such infants and varies in relation to the environmental temperature. It is necessary to assist the infant to maintain an optimum body temperature which for the low birth weight infant is approximately 36° to 37°C (rectal). The general care of these infants requires the use of a special incubator which can be heated to high temperatures with raised humidity levels (Figs 2.1–2.4) and with this method the infant is usually partially unclothed. If an incubator is not available maintenance of body temperature requires that the infant be adequately clothed and the room in which the infant is nursed is heated to a temperature of approximately 24° to 26·6°C. The atmosphere should also be humid to a level of 65 to 70 per cent saturation and even higher. Special care units for low birth weight infants should have available special low-reading thermometers which record lower temperature levels than the usual clinical thermometers.

Establishment and maintenance of respiratory function. To initiate respiratory function, which is poor in these infants, the usual methods are used such as gentle clearing of the air passages and maintaining a warm atmosphere. Oxygen may be required. Neonatal asphyxia is discussed in another section of this book.

Once respiratory function has been established its maintenance requires much care and the use of oxygen may be necessary. The indication for oxygen therapy in these infants is the presence of cyanosis, and the amount of oxygen which should be given is the least amount which will prevent the baby from becoming cyanosed. It is useful to determine and monitor the arterial blood oxygen saturation and in advanced special care centres these arterial blood oxygen concentrations are measured and used in controlling oxygen administration to these infants. A transcutaneous oxygen monitor is becoming available for use in these special care units. Arterial oxygen tension (Po_2) between 60 and 90 mmHg is necessary for normal tissue oxygenation. The concentration of oxygen administered to these infants should seldom exceed 40 per cent but higher concentrations may be necessary to correct hypoxia. In this connection it is essential that an oxygen analyser and monitor should be available in every centre caring for the low birth weight infant so that oxygen concentration readings can be taken to prevent the overoxygenation of these babies. Electronic

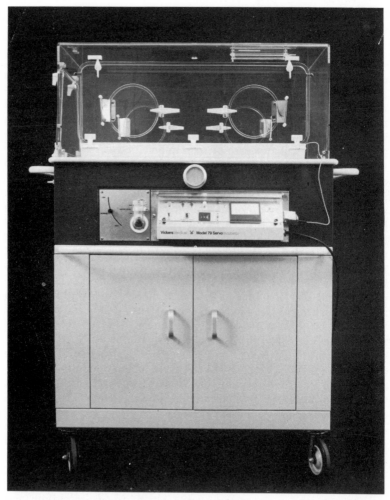

Fig. 2.1 Vickers model 79 servo control incubator. (*By courtesy of Vickers Ltd.*)

monitoring equipment may be useful in the general management of the sick infant and allow for the early warning of complications. The parameters that can be monitored include the ECG, pulse, respiration, temperature and blood pressure levels. Another useful and simpler method of monitoring respiration and allowing for early warning of apnoea is the apnoea alarm mattress (Fig. 2.5) where the infant lies on a special sectional air-bed which has the ability to electrically detect cross-flow air passage in the mattress and will sound an alarm if the mattress fails to detect movement such as by apnoea. As mentioned before, the infant should be nursed in a humid atmosphere.

Prevention of infection. These infants have lowered resistance to infection, and it is most important to prevent any likelihood of such a happening. The facts are probably related to the relative deficiency of immunoglobulins at birth and this is discussed in another section of

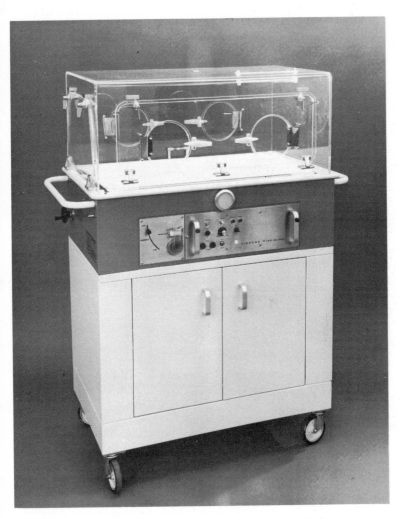

Fig. 2.2 Vickers 'Five-Nine' incubator. (*By courtesy of Vickers Ltd.*)

this book. Only persons who deal with the infant should have contact with it, and they should, of course, themselves be free from infections such as the common cold, diarrhoea, sore throat or skin infections and also other infections. No visitors should be allowed and all those who deal with the infant must be adequately gowned. It is absolutely essential that careful hand washing be undertaken by all those handling these infants and the use of disposable items should be encouraged. Some authorities have advised the use of human immunoglobulin or

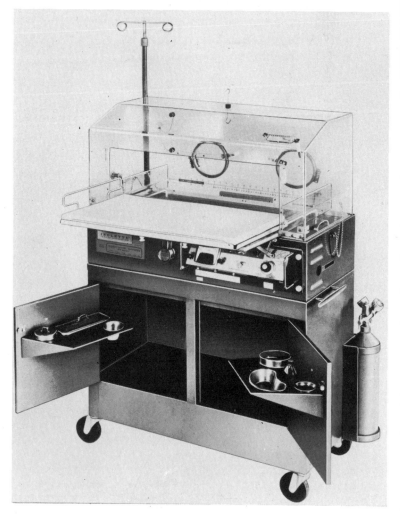

Fig. 2.3 Air-Shields Isolette intensive care infant incubator.

penicillin or other antibiotic on a prophylactic basis to prevent infection in certain infants, but this is not generally supported.

Feeding. These infants should be handled very gently. It is necessary for the initial feeding of the low birth weight infant to start early and

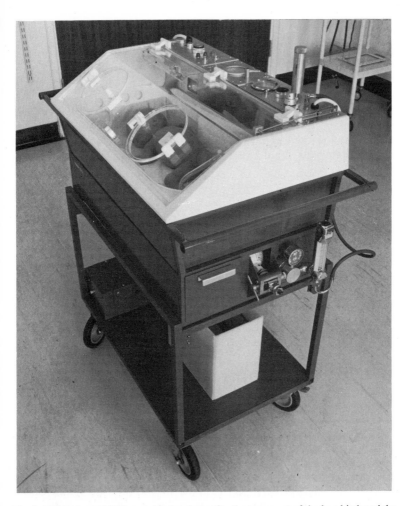

Fig. 2.4 Vickers model 77 portable incubator for the transport of the low birth weight infant under sheltered and warm conditions. (*By courtesy of Vickers Ltd.*)

as soon as conveniently possible after birth. This early feeding is necessary to avoid hypoglycaemia (low blood glucose) occurring but proper care must be taken to prevent aspiration with subsequent asphyxial attacks. Breast milk may be used but usually feeding is started with small amounts of sterile water followed by glucose water at three-hourly intervals, the amount depending on the size of the infant. This is followed by giving expressed breast milk; the quantity of the breast milk should then be gradually increased so that by approximately the tenth to fourteenth day after birth the infant is receiving feeds in the required amounts.

In discussing feeding the following points must be answered:

(a) What feed to offer
(b) The quantity of feeds to offer
(c) The frequency of feeding
(d) The method of feeding

Breast milk is the best feed for infant feeding including the low birth weight infant, but if this is not available modified cow's milk preparations may be used. The amount of fluid that the child requires is approximately 200 ml of breast milk per kg bodyweight per 24 hours, or

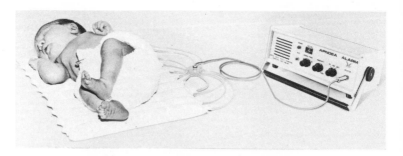

Fig. 2.5 Apnoea alarm mattress. (*By courtesy of Vickers Ltd.*)

135 kilocalories per kg bodyweight. Some authorities advise a higher calorific intake for these infants, but this would require additions to the breast milk and is not generally supported. The frequency of feeding depends on the size of the child, the smaller the infant the more frequent feeds it should have. The larger infants may do adequately with three-hourly feeds through the 24 hours, and the smaller infants two-hourly feeds by day and three-hourly by night. The method of feeding again depends on the size of the infant. Those infants that are big enough and can adequately suck and swallow may be fed by bottle with a small teat; the small infant must be fed by oesphageal tube using a disposable plastic feeding tube which is also useful if left *in situ* for anything up to three or four days.

Miscellaneous. Vitamin K_1 should be given soon after birth to ensure an adequate prothrombin level in the blood to prevent haemorrhage. A small dose is sufficient for this prophylactic use and large doses should not be used as evidence has accumulated that excessive use of vitamin K may increase the occurrence of jaundice in some cases. The fat-soluble vitamins A and D may be started by mouth during the third or fourth week by giving approximately 3000 units of vitamin A and 1000 vitamin D daily. Vitamin C (ascorbic acid) should also be started at this stage in an amount of 25 to 50 mg daily. These vitamins are best given in an aqueous solution and many multivitamin preparations are available. Iron is also necessary as the preterm infant has not a sufficient iron store to support haemopoiesis (red cell formation); iron should be administered by mouth from the fourth week in an easily absorbed preparation.

Dangers

The low birth weight infant is liable to many dangers; many of these infants that die do so in the first 24 hours after birth. They are likely to develop haemorrhage because of the fragility of their blood vessels. Intracranial haemorrhage is very common and in the small infant this may be intraventricular where the cause is probably hypoxia and may be related to disseminated intravascular coagulation. These infants are likely to develop asphyxial states and the idiopathic respiratory distress. syndrome (IRDS) with hyaline membrane (Fig. 2.6) particularly affects the low birth weight infant. In these cases of the hyaline membrane

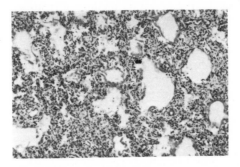

Fig. 2.6 Histopathological section of the lung suitably stained to show hyaline membranes lining the air sacs in hyaline membrane disease.

syndrome, in addition to the asphyxial state produced, there is also the danger of acidosis with its grave consequences. This syndrome has a high mortality (up to 40 per cent) and much research has been undertaken in an attempt to elucidate the possible aetiological factors. It is known that this idiopathic respiratory distress syndrome with hyaline membrane affects particularly the preterm infant, infants born of diabetic mothers and the infant born by caesarean section (where the cause, however, probably lies more with the indication for the caesarean section rather than the section itself).

Various causes were thought to be important in the aetiology of this disease and an important factor is the deficiency or inactivation of surface active material or surfactant in the lung which tends to lower surface tension in the alveoli of the lungs. The hyaline membrane has fibrin as a constituent, this having its origin as a transudation from the pulmonary capillary vessels into the alveoli. The major problem of the low birth weight preterm infant is this idiopathic respiratory distress syndrome with hyaline membrane formation and it accounts for a high proportion of deaths of these infants in the first few days after birth. The clinical features of this condition include severe chest retraction, subcostal, substernal and intercostal recession, expiratory grunt with diminished air entry developing usually some time after birth and persisting longer than three hours. The respiratory rate markedly increases and apnoeic attacks often complicate the picture; cardio-vascular signs may be found with hepatic enlargement, hypotension (low blood pressure) and oedema. Radiologically the lung fields show a granular appearance with a clear outline of the trachea and bronchi ('air bronchogram'). A system of assessing severity by grading chest retractions and other signs have been devised by Silverman and Anderson. These infants have been shown to develop a severe respiratory acidosis and an approach on the management in relation to the control of these biochemical changes, as originally suggested by Usher in Canada, is a necessary method of treatment. This requires that the blood pH and the blood gases be regularly measured in addition to other biochemical estimations and the therapy of intravenous dextrose solution infusion with sodium bicarbonate be administered. THAM (tris-hydroxymethylaminomethane) has also been used to combat acidosis. The biochemical estimations can be performed on small quantities of blood with the Astrup micro equipment or similar apparatus. Antibiotics are necessary and controlled oxygen therapy is essential with the high humidity in which these infants are nursed. The respiratory function may have to be assisted with the use of various methods such as continuous positive airway pressure (CPAP) using the Gregory box (Fig. 2.7), or intermittent positive pressure respiration (IPPR) using a suitable ventilator or continuous negative pressure (CNP). The results of treatment are improving with the better and more rational care that is being given to these infants.

Infection is particularly likely to affect low birth weight infants especially the preterm, and its prevention has been discussed. The deficiency of certain immunoglobulins may explain the lowered resistance to infection. An ophthalmic condition, retrolental fibroplasia, which may progress to blindness is known to occur in the preterm infant. It is known that this condition is related to the administration of excess oxygen to these infants causing vascular changes to the retinal blood vessels. With this knowledge this preventable condition has become less common with improved control of oxygen administration. Where the possibility exists it is essential that ophthalmoscopic examination of the fundi of these infants be regularly and carefully done and there is a method of indirect ophthalmoscopy available for this purpose. As mentioned before, oxygen administration to these infants must be carefully controlled and should only be given to those infants that require it; an oxygen analyser and monitor should

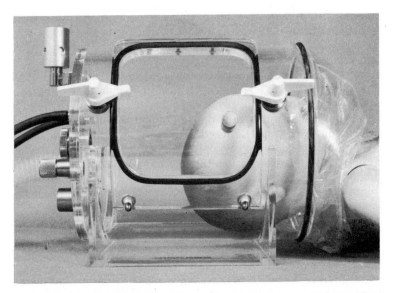

Fig. 2.7 Vickers continuous positive airway pressure (CPAP) system (Gregory box). (*By courtesy of Vickers Ltd.*)

be available in every centre caring for these infants, so that regular oxygen concentrations can be monitored. Cyanotic attacks are likely to affect these infants and may be associated with overdistension of the stomach after too large a feed. Oedema is likely to occur in these small infants and this may be associated with immature kidney function, low blood protein levels or by allowing the child to become too cold. Neonatal cold injury (hypothermia) is a possible complicating condition in the low birth weight infant and this is discussed in another section. Late conditions which may affect these infants are anaemia and the deficiency disease of rickets. These small infants have a high incidence of jaundice and in some cases this may become severe by the fifth to the seventh day and lead to bilirubin encephalopathy (kernicterus) in the same way as certain cases of haemolytic disease of the newborn are complicated by this severe and often fatal condition. This is discussed in more detail in another section. The low birth weight for gestation infant ('small-for-dates') is especially liable to develop hypoglycaemia and this serious complication must be carefully controlled as it is possible that brain damage may occur with these episodes of hypoglycaemia. In those infants that are susceptible to this condition developing it is essential that regular blood glucose levels be estimated and for rapid results use may be made of a glucose oxidase test paper (Dextrostix). Early feeding is useful in the prevention of hypoglycaemia and if the condition occurs treatment with intravenous dextrose solutions should be used; the corticosteroids may also be useful. Frequent intramuscular injections in the neonatal period, especially to the low birth weight infant, may cause fibrosis of the quadriceps muscle which may lead to contracture of the muscle with limitation of knee flexion in later childhood.

An unusual complication affecting the more immature infants of less than 32 weeks gestation is interstitial pulmonary fibrosis of prematurity (Wilson-Mikity syndrome, or the bubbly lung syndrome). The clinical symptoms usually develop some time after birth and are insidious in their onset. Respiratory difficulty with attacks of apnoea, cyanosis and collapse occur; abdominal distension and rib fractures are other features. The diagnosis may be confirmed by radiological examination which shows diffuse lung changes with small rounded clear radio-translucent areas. There is a tendency towards improvement in this condition but respiratory failure may occur.

Prevention of respiratory distress syndrome (RDS)

The most rational approach to the prevention of this condition would be to prevent premature labour but until that can happen the respiratory distress syndrome will continue to be a major hazard. There has been speculation from animal studies that the administration of hydrocortisone may induce the production of surfactant. The amniotic fluid may be tested for information in relation to the production of pulmonary surfactant and an estimation is made of the lecithin:sphingomyelin ratio and the concentration of lecithin and these investigations appear to correlate with the subsequent condition of the infant. A simplified modification of this test in relation to the amniotic fluid forming a stable foam is available but false results may be obtained. A positive result indicates maturity of the foetal lung with less likelihood of the respiratory distress syndrome affecting the newborn infant after birth.

Prognosis

The immediate prognosis of these infants depends on the gestational period and the birth weight and it is logical that the longer the period of gestation and the heavier the child the better is the prognosis for immediate survival. The immediate prognosis is also affected by the cause, if known, of the premature labour; where the cause is due to maternal illness the prognosis will always be worse than for other causes. The ultimate prognosis is a debatable question but there is little doubt that many of these low birth weight infants achieve normality both mentally and physically.

3. Breast Feeding

There is no doubt that the best food for infants is human breast milk. Unfortunately there has been a tendency for breast feeding to become less commonly practised in many countries and this fact cannot be too strongly deprecated. There is convincing evidence that breast feeding has many advantages to both infant and mother and is a safeguard against a variety of conditions which are important to the infant's future. It is difficult to define clearly the causes of the lowered incidence of breast feeding but there is little doubt that social factors play a large part. In certain cases they are related to the mother having to return to work or her household duties and associated worries soon after the parturition period. Certain mothers require more assistance than others in establishing successful breast feeding. An increased knowledge of the benefits of breast feeding and better propaganda in its favour would do much to lessen the lowering incidence of breast feeding. Apart from changes in the pattern of life as a cause of the changing attitudes to breast feeding the promotion of artificial feeds is probably also a factor.

Advantages

Breast milk is sterile, taken at the correct temperature, and has an adequate constitution for the optimum growth of the baby. There is little doubt that infants do better when breast fed and are brought into the closest contact with the mother, who is most concerned with the welfare of her baby, and this satisfactory relationship between mother and child is of lasting psychological benefit to both. Feeding difficulties happen far more frequently in the artificially fed infant than in the breast fed. Breast feeding does not need as much attention as artificial feeding and is more economic.

Deficiency states of infants are less common in the breast-fed infant and acute diarrhoeal disorders of infancy occur far less often in the breast-fed infant. There is the possibility that allergic patterns may be laid down by early contact of the infant with proteins and other substances in artificial feeds and that this possibility may be lessened in the infant wholly breast fed in the early days after birth.

Contraindications

There are some contraindications to breast feeding. These include conditions such as active pulmonary tuberculosis in the mother which would expose the child to the danger of contracting tuberculosis at a most vulnerable age; furthermore, breast feeding in these cases would also be detrimental to the health of the mother. In certain circumstances where nutritional problems may arise in the non-breast-fed infant in underdeveloped countries, it may be necessary to allow for a continuation of breast feeding where the mother is actively treated for her tuberculosis infection; a useful measure in such cases is to give these infants prophylactic isoniazid (INAH). Mental illness in the mother such as puerperal psychosis is also a contraindication in certain circumstances as this condition may expose the child to physical injury. Epilepsy may also be a contraindication in certain circumstances. A further contraindication is another pregnancy developing in the lactating mother. Acute illness in the mother also serves as a contraindication and chronic illness such as heart or renal disease may be a possible contraindication depending on the extent of the disability. Various local conditions of the breast, such as retracted or cracked nipples, might be a temporary disability until cured when breast feeding can restart provided that the milk supply has been maintained. Another temporary contraindication is a breast abscess. Breast malignancy is a definite reason for discontinuing breast feeding. Certain conditions in the infant such as severe cleft palate and harelip may preclude breast feeding and in the low birth weight infant expressed breast milk should be used.

Preparation of the mother

It is essential that the mother be prepared properly in the antenatal period and this must include the psychological attitudes that are adopted. The diet of these mothers must be adequate and must contain sufficient protein and vitamins and other essentials. The breast and nipples should be prepared for breast feeding in the last trimester of the pregnancy and abnormalities such as retraction of the nipples should be treated with a breast shield. It is essential that the adequate diet be continued during lactation. In the early days of lactation it is essential that engorgement and congestion of the breasts should be prevented. There is little doubt that the strongest stimulus to adequate breast milk in a mother is the suckling of the baby and the regular complete emptying of the breast. Soon after birth the breast secretes a yellowish rather thick fluid called colostrum. Colostrum has approximately five times the amount of protein of breast milk, twice the amount of salts and half the amount of carbohydrate and fat. Full lactation of the breast takes place in about three days when the colostrum is replaced by breast milk. Colostrum appears to carry immune antibodies to the infant and has also been said to act as a laxative thereby helping the infant to pass meconium.

Composition of breast milk

Breast milk is made up of:

1. Protein, in a percentage of 1·25. This protein consists of two parts of lactalbumin and one part of caseinogen. The lactalbumin is rich in the essential amino acids and is therefore an important constituent of the milk.
2. Carbohydrate, in a percentage of 7·25. This carbohydrate is lactose, and milk is in fact the only natural source of this carbohydrate.
3. Fat, in a percentage of 3·5. The fat in breast milk is present in small globules in a fine emulsion.
4. Salts, in a percentage of 0·2. These salts include sodium (18 mg per 100 ml), potassium (55 mg per 100 ml), chlorides (43 mg per 100 ml), calcium (33 mg per 100 ml), phosphate (15 mg per 100 ml), magnesium (4 mg per 100 ml), iron (0·15 mg per 100 ml), copper (40 μg per 100 ml). Iron is present in a slightly higher quantity than in cow's milk (0·10 mg per 100 ml) but still insufficient for the needs of the baby.
5. Vitamins are present in an amount depending on the nutrition and diet of the mother with the following approximate content: vitamin A, 200 i.u. per 100 ml; vitamin C, 5 mg per 100 ml; and vitamin D, 2 i.u. per 100 ml.
6. Water.

Technique of breast feeding

The infant must be held in a comfortable position with no obstruction to the breathing. The infant may be put to the breast within a few hours after birth, usually within six hours. This feeding may be continued four hourly on the second day and then four hourly or three hourly depending on the size of the child. The infant of about 3·5 kg or over usually does well on a four-hourly schedule. The ultimate quantitative requirements of the infant are approximately 150 to 165 ml of breast milk per kg bodyweight per day, or 110 kilocalories (kcal) per kg per day. (One hundred ml of breast milk provides approximately 67 kcal of energy.)

The infant should be fed for not longer than 15 to 20 minutes, and each breast can be offered in turn allowing $7\frac{1}{2}$ to 10 minutes at each side. It is important to realise that the infant receives about three-quarters of the feed in the first five minutes but the breast should be completely emptied as the hindmilk, or 'strippings', contain a higher fat content than the foremilk.

The output of milk from the breast is highest at the first feed of the day and lowest at the midday or two o'clock feed. The other feeds give less milk than the first feed and more than the midday feed and this fact is of importance in test weighing an infant to determine the daily intake. The procedure of test weighing an infant should be done over a 24 hour period to include all feeds taken in that time. The baby should be weighed before and after each feed with the same clothing and must include any stools or urine passed during that particular feed. In the first few days after birth an infant loses weight but regains the birth weight by approximately the tenth day after birth. From that time the weight gain is approximately 20 g per day so that the birth weight is doubled by the fifth month. From that time the weight gain is at a slower rate so that the birth weight is trebled at approximately 1 year of age. When the infant is about 4 months old the diet must be supplemented, but it is necessary to stress that the early introduction of cereals and other solid foods to the diet of babies before about 4 months of age should be discouraged. The diet is supplemented in order to get the child used to different tastes, to develop the skill of dealing with and swallowing solid sieved foods, and also to supply iron and roughage. Vegetables, egg yolk, fruit, cereals, meat and other sieved foods may be slowly added and eventually replacing the breast feeds.

Problems of breast feeding

Engorgement and congestion. The engorgement of the breasts especially in primigravida is not uncommon and is associated with congestion and there is associated pain. This condition may develop quickly and often appears about the third or fourth day after birth. It is due to the failure to remove the breast secretions associated with some obstruction to its outlet in the nipple ducts. Adequate care of the breasts in the antenatal period is the best preventative method. The distension should be relieved by manual expression and temporary reduction of the mother's fluid intake. The judicious use of small doses of stilboestrol under strict control may be necessary to relieve pain. When the ducts are patent and the tension is relieved the infant should be put back to the breast.

Failure of suckling. A cleft palate and harelip may be present and feeding may also be hindered in the low birth weight infant. Nasal obstruction or some infection of the mouth such as thrush may also cause a failure of normal suckling. A severe congenital cardiac lesion may prevent adequate suckling as may other causes of breathlessness. Retracted nipples may also be a factor in preventing proper breast feeding.

Underfeeding. This is an important cause of a failure to thrive and at first the weight gain becomes slow then the weight remains stationary and eventually there is a loss of weight. The infant becomes irritable with excessive crying especially at night. There is air swallowing and consequent vomiting and constipation develops, but on occasion the infant may pass frequent small, green stools (hunger or starvation stools). The diagnosis is confirmed by test weighing and the amount of underfeeding may be replaced by a complementary feed by which the infant is offered an extra artificial feed after a breast feed. This is in contrast to supplementary feeding where an entire breast feed is replaced by an artificial feed.

Overfeeding. This is a very rare occurrence and may occur more often in the early months. There is a rapid gain in weight at first with some regurgitation of the feed. Frequent loose stools are passed but these are of a normal yellow colour. The diagnosis is confirmed by test weighing and the treatment requires either offering water before the feed or altering a three-hourly schedule to a four-hourly one.

Drugs in breast milk. Various medicines which the lactating mother takes may be excreted in her milk. The anticoagulants, antithyroid drugs, salicylates, oral contraceptives and the corticosteroids are excreted. Excessive smoking or alcohol may affect the infant. The barbiturate drugs may be excreted in breast milk to produce drowsiness in the feeding infant. The sulphonamides, penicillin and other antibiotics, and the antihistamine drugs are excreted, but not usually sufficiently to affect the child. The anthracene purgatives such as senna and cascara may be excreted in sufficient quantity to affect the infant and produce loose stools. It is probably unwise for lactating mothers to take the newer drugs unless definitely indicated.

Demand feeding. This type of feeding requires that the infant is offered a feed on demand, usually by crying. This method has much to commend it and is associated with an easier and more permissive attitude to infant feeding and is in contrast to the rigid schedule feeding of infants by the clock. Successful demand feeding requires proper appreciation of this method by the mother and it is often found in actual practice that feeding by demand eventually approximates to a fairly regular feeding schedule.

4. Artificial Feeding

In many countries artificial feeding has become common although over the years many cyclical changes have happened. At one time great emphasis was placed on clear definitions of infant feeding mixtures in relation to the precise concentration of the constituents of feeds. This has also related to the calorific values required for the growing infant. Since that time many changes have taken place and the tendency has been towards an easier and more permissive approach to infant feeding, but there is fortunately again an interest developing in relation to nutrition and the possible effects on the future wellbeing of the individual. It is important and necessary for persons dealing with the care of the normal infant and its feeding, when breast feeding is not available, to have knowledge of the composition and other aspects of the principal substitute feed which is cow's milk.

Composition of cow's milk

Carbohydrate is present as lactose in a percentage of 4·5. As mentioned previously the only natural source of lactose is in milk. Fat is present in an average amount of about 3·5 per cent, but this amount varies with the breed of animal, the Jersey cow for example having a higher fat content. The fat of cow's milk consists of the triglycerides of the non-volatile acids and also of volatile acids. The fat globules are large and coarse, unlike the fine globules of breast milk, and the fat readily decomposes under the influence of light, oxygen and bacteria. Protein is present in cow's milk in a percentage of 3·5 and this protein consists of casein and lactalbumin in a proportion of five parts casein to one part lactalbumin. This differs from the proportions in breast milk where it is present as two-thirds lactalbumin and one-third casein. The protein of cow's milk produces a thick, coarse curd in the baby's stomach, unlike the fine, softly textured curd of breast milk. There are various methods of modifying the protein of cow's milk in order to make it more digestible, and these include dilution with water, boiling and drying.

Vitamins. The vitamin content of cow's milk depends to some extent on the care and nutrition of the animal. Vitamin A is present in approximately 150 i.u. per 100 ml, vitamin C in an amount of 1·5 mg per 100 ml, and vitamin D as approximately 1·3 i.u. per 100 ml. The vitamin C is destroyed by boiling or pasteurisation.

Salts. Salts in cow's milk are present in an amount of 0·7 per cent.

The sodium content is 58 mg per 100 ml, potassium 138 mg, chloride 103 mg, calcium 125 mg, magnesium 12 mg, phosphate 96 mg, iron 0·10 mg, copper 30 μg per 100 ml. The iron content is insufficient for the needs of the infant. The calcium and phosphate levels are present in cow's milk in an approximate ratio of 1·35: 1 in contrast to the ratio in breast milk of 2: 1. This fact favours higher blood phosphate levels and disturbed calcium absorption and this may lead to hypo-calcaemic tetany in the immediate neonatal period. This situation appears to be avoidable if the ratio of calcium and phosphate is closer to that in human breast milk, and modifications to artificial feed in this direction has taken place. Neonatal tetany requires as treatment the administration of calcium. Another type of tetany may be associated with low magnesium blood levels with normal calcium and phosphate levels and this condition requires the administration of magnesium. Some of these modified artificial feeds are available as prepacked 'ready to feed' liquid milks and this has simplified feeding but has the distinct disadvantage of lowering the interest in breast feeding.

Bacteriology of milk

Milk may be contaminated by various methods and may contain a variety of bacteria. The origin of these bacteria may be in the cow itself or from its skin. Bacterial infection may also arise from the hands and throat of the milker, from the utensils in which the milk is placed, from the dairy, or by contamination by flies in the home. Cow's milk has been the origin of epidemics of typhoid fever and also of strepto-coccal infections. Brucellosis and acute infantile diarrhoea may also have its origin from infected cow's milk. Finally tuberculosis may have its origin in cow's milk.

Types of milk available for infant feeding

Fluid milk. This is available as raw, pasteurised, tuberculin tested and homogenised and sterilised. The pasteurisation process implies heating milk to a temperature of about 65°C for half an hour and rapidly cooling to a temperature below 7·2°C. Another more generally used method of pasteurisation is the high temperature short time method (HTST) where the high temperature is 73°C for 15 seconds and is followed by rapid cooling. This milk should not contain more than 100,000 bacteria per ml. Whenever milk is used in artificial feeding it must be boiled for a period of about two to three minutes in order to destroy any bacteria present. This process and also pasteurisation destroys the vitamin C content of the milk but this is of no consequence in feeding provided this lack of vitamin C is made good.

Dried milks. Dried milks are produced by various methods such as the spray method whereby milk is forced through fine jets under pressure into a heated chamber to drive off the water and allow the powdered milk to drop to the floor of the chamber. The roller drying method requires the fluid milk to be poured on to rotating hot rollers from which the water is driven off and the powder left attached to the roller from which it is scraped. Freeze drying is another method. The spray-dried preparation is usually available for use in infant feeding and different types of dried milks are available. These types include:

1. Unmodified dried milk powders such as Cow and Gate Babymilk 2, Ostermilk Two and National Dried Milk are not recommended for infant feeding.
2. Modified dried milk powders some with the addition of carbo-hydrate such as Cow and Gate Babymilk Plus, Cow and Gate Trufood, Ostermilk Complete Formula, Cow and Gate Premium Babyfood.
3. Dried milk powders where the fat is replaced by other fats such as Cow and Gate V Formula, SMA, and SMA S26 (Gold Cap). Dried milks are widely used in infant feeding and have the advantage that they are sterile and have a constant composition.
4. Modified 'ready to feed' liquid preparations include Cow and Gate, Ostermilk and SMA and are available in 120 ml and 100 ml con-tainers. They are extremely useful for hospital use but as mentioned previously have the disadvantage of possibly discouraging attempts to establish successful breast feeding. An added disadvantage is that mothers do not obtain the experience of preparing artificial feeds for use on their discharge from maternity units.
5. Evaporated milks are available in various types where the water is removed by heating the milk *in vacuo* under pressure so as to leave more concentrated milk preparations. There are modified evaporated preparations available such as SMA (Gold Cap) and also un-modified such as Carnation (not recommended) which must have water added to reconstitute to ordinary cow's milk. Sweetened condensed milk is a concentrated milk preparation with added sucrose which should not be encouraged in infant feeding except as a temporary measure, as it leads to flabbiness with a tendency to develop obesity and rickets.

Method of calculating infant feeds

Certain principles must be remembered although there are no hard and fast rules to apply to the calculation of infant feeds. The principles include the fluid requirements of the baby and also the caloric require-ments. An infant needs about 150 to 165 ml of fluid per kg bodyweight per day, or 100 to 110 kilocalories per kg per day. Cow's milk has a calorific value of 66 per 100 ml and 4 g of cane sugar provides 15 kilo-calories. As a general rule it may be said that the child in the first two weeks of life will do well on slightly more than half-strength cow's milk with added sugar while from the second week onward until about the fourth month the requirement is approximately 100 ml of boiled cow's milk per kg bodyweight per day. This amount must be diluted with water, which has been boiled, to make up the required amount of 150 ml per kg bodyweight per day. Sugar is added to the feed in the form of cane sugar (sucrose). The various equivalents in modified low solute milk preparations either dried or evaporated are preferably used in place of fluid milk. As an example of calculating a feed for a normal 5 kg infant this would require 150 ml of fluid per day multiplied five times, i.e. 750 ml of fluid in the day. The cow's milk requirement of this amount would be 100 ml per kilo, i.e. 500 ml of cow's milk per day. To this amount water must be added to bring it to the required amount of 750 ml, i.e. 250 ml of water must be added. In addition sugar is added to the whole day's feed in an amount of approximately 30 g.

As a general rule an infant of approximately 3·5 kg or over would require five feeds in the day, therefore this infant of 5 kg would need five feeds of 150 ml per feed giving him the required 750 ml in the day. These feeds are usually given at approximately 6.00 a.m., 10.00 a.m., 2.00 p.m., 6.00 p.m. and 10.00 p.m.

The artificially fed infant must also have vitamins supplied and these include ascorbic acid (vitamin C) which can be provided in orange juice, and vitamins A and D in a suitable preparation. There are many good proprietary multivitamin preparations available which supply the vitamin needs of infants. In relation to the introduction of solids this should not start before about the fourth month after birth and cereal foods should not be added to the bottled milk feeds. The early introduction of solids has led to problems in relation to overweight infants and should be discouraged. In relation to this aspect mothers should also be advised not to add sugar or salt to the solid foods in the infant diet.

Preparation of artificial feeds
Bottles and teats. The Soxhlet type of bottle with one open end is in general use in infant feeding and has the advantage that the feed may be sterilised in the bottle itself and that the whole day's feed may be made up and stored together. The teat should have an adequately sized hole which allows the infant to feed without great difficulty. If the hole is too small it may be enlarged by using a red-hot needle. The teats and bottle should be cleansed and sterilised after each feed and for this purpose a special solution of a chlorine-containing substance (Milton, Nursery Hysan) may be used; boiling as a means of sterilisation can also be used, and the bottles and teats should then be immersed and left in cold sterile water until used. The hands of the person feeding the infant should be washed before handling the feed or utensils. Dried milks are mixed to a paste with cold boiled water after which hot boiled water is added to the required quantity.

Timing of feeds
The infant should take the complete feed in about 15 minutes without

great effort. He should be allowed to break wind halfway through the feed and after completion. As mentioned before, infants of approximately 3·5 kg and over usually require five feeds in the 24 hours and those under this weight six feeds; the demand method of feeding usually approximates to this type of plan and also, as mentioned previously, vitamins must be given to all artificially fed infants.

The introduction of solids to the milk diet at about 4 months of age requires the addition of various sieved foods such as vegetables, fruit, fish and meat and also egg yolk and cereals. These are necessary to prevent the child developing anaemia, to get him used to different tastes, to provide increased bulk, and to allow the infant to become used to the cup and spoon and to acquire the new skills of dealing with and swallowing solid foods.

5. Neonatal Paediatrics

The neonatal mortality rate, as defined in a previous section, is the number of deaths in the first month of life per 1000 live births. In recent years many countries of the world have achieved a tremendous reduction of the infant mortality rate, but only to a lesser extent of the neonatal mortality rate. Most neonatal deaths are due to prematurity and low birth weight, birth trauma, infection, asphyxial states and congenital abnormalities. The majority of neonatal deaths occur during the first week of life (in some series up to 75 per cent). Of these deaths about a half take place on the first day of life. Affections of the newborn might be considered under the following sections:

Congenital anomalies
Conditions directly due to the birth process
Asphyxia and anoxia
Infection
Haemorrhagic conditions
Neonatal jaundice
Miscellaneous conditions, such as inanition fever or dehydration fever of the newborn and mastitis neonatorum

CONGENITAL ANOMALIES

Congenital abnormalities cause a fair proportion of infant deaths (Figs 5.1 to 5.19). Much attention has been focused on the possible causes of congenital abnormalities. This interest was stimulated by the discovery by Gregg in Australia of the relationship between rubella (German measles) affecting the mother in the first few weeks of pregnancy, and congenital abnormalities developing in the child. It has been suggested that the presence of a single umbilical artery instead of the normal two may be associated with a higher incidence of congenital anomalies. The following are some of the possible causes:

1. Virus infections—rubella
2. Irradiation—X-rays
3. Diet (?)·
4. Heredity
5. Position of foetus *in utero*
6. Drugs

27

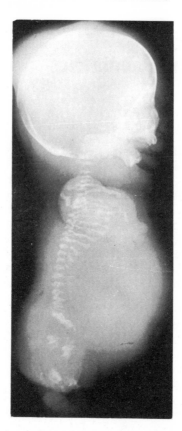

Fig. 5.1 Radiograph of a grossly abnormal stillborn infant with phocomelia where the hands and feet are attached to the trunk by a single irregular bone (lateral view).

Virus infections of pregnant women. Rubella occurring during early pregnancy can cause congenital abnormality in the child, especially congenital cataracts (Fig. 5.11), congenital deafness, congenital heart disease such as a patent ductus arteriosus or an atrial septal defect and mental retardation (with or without microcephaly) and other abnormalities. The association of maternal rubella and congenital infection of the foetus is discussed in another section of this book. Other virus infections such as mumps and influenza have also been reported as causing congenital abnormality in the developing foetus.

Excessive *irradiation* during early pregnancy may affect the developing embryo.

Dietetic factors are also possibly involved, but there is no proof of this in man, although some congenital abnormalities have been produced in the offspring of pregnant rats fed on a deficient diet.

Heredogenetic causes.

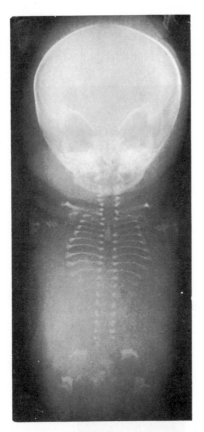

Fig. 5.2 Anteroposterior radiograph of the same case as Fig. 5.1.

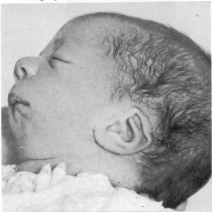

Fig. 5.3 Micrognathos (recession of the chin due to hypoplasia of the mandible). This condition may be associated with cyanotic attacks in the newborn due to recession of the tongue (Pierre-Robin syndrome).

Abnormal position of the developing foetus in utero may produce orthopaedic congenital abnormalities such as club feet and valgus deformities of the feet. Amniotic bands might also produce abnormalities.

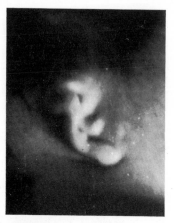

Fig. 5.4 Congenital abnormality of the external ear.

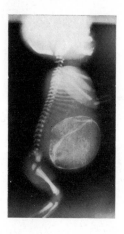

Fig. 5.5 X-ray of a stillborn child with a calcified urachal cyst.

With the increasing use of new *drugs* in pregnancy it has been suggested that congenital abnormalities of the foetus might be produced. A sedative drug, thalidomide (Distaval) has been withdrawn from medical usage as it has been shown to produce severe congenital abnormalities, especially aplasia and hypoplasia of the extremities (amelia and phocomelia—Figs 5.1 and 5.2) and malformations of other organs.

CONDITIONS DIRECTLY DUE TO THE BIRTH PROCESS

Birth trauma

Birth trauma should be considered in relation to the various parts of the infant that might be injured.

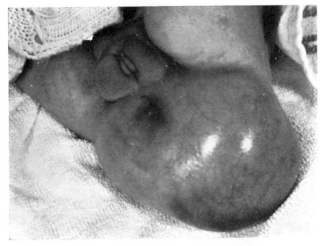

Fig. 5.6 Sacrococcygeal tumour (teratoma) in a newborn female infant. (Successfully removed.) (*By courtesy from Lannon & Smith: 'South African Medical Journal'.*)

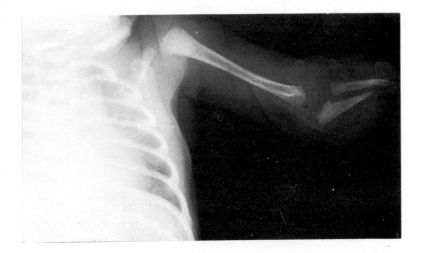

Fig. 5.7 X-ray of the left upper limb in a newborn child with congenital amputation of the forearm.

Cranial injuries

There may be trauma to the skull bones and their coverings and also injury to the brain itself.

Caput succedaneum. This is a swelling affecting the head of the newly born infant and is due to an effusion of fluid into the skin and subcutaneous tissues of the presenting part after birth. This swelling is of little consequence and disappears quite rapidly.

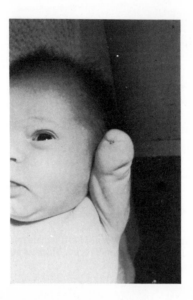

Fig. 5.8 Congenital amputation of the forearm.

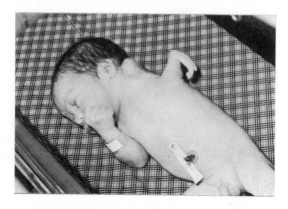

Fig. 5.9 Congenital amputation of left upper limb with a supernumerary limb attached to the chest wall.

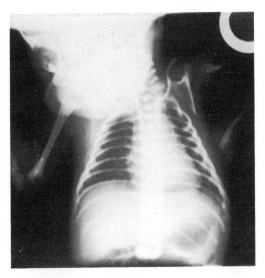

Fig. 5.10 X-ray of same infant as Fig. 5.9.

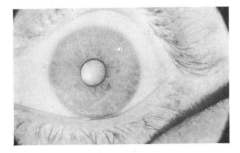

Fig. 5.11 A cataract in the lens of the eye as seen in bilateral congenital cataract caused by rubella in early pregnancy.

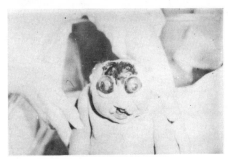

Fig. 5.12 Anencephaly with cleft lip and palate.

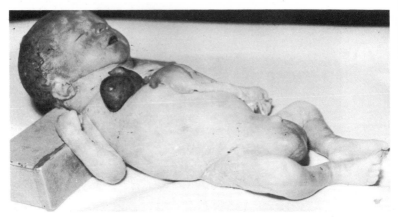

Fig. 5.13 Ectopia cordis.

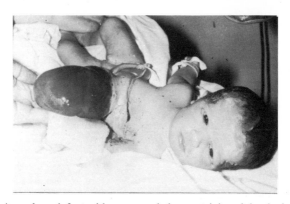

Fig. 5.14 A newborn infant with an exomphalos containing abdominal contents.

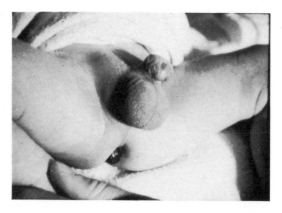

Fig. 5.15 Hypospadias.

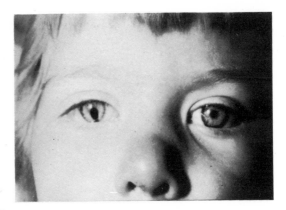

Fig. 5.16 Right coloboma of the iris.

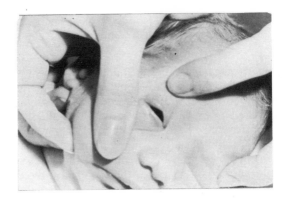

Fig. 5.17 Coloboma of the right upper eyelid.

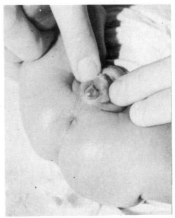

Fig. 5.18 Vaginal cyst; simulating an imperforate hymen with a hydrocolpos.

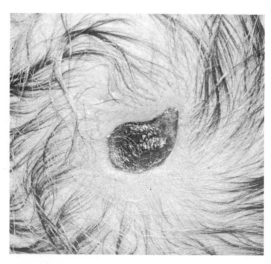

Fig. 5.19 Congenital skin defect of scalp.

Cephalhaematoma (Figs 5.20 and 5.21). This consists of an effusion of blood between a cranial bone and its periosteum. It is usually apparent on the second or third day after birth and consists of a tense cystic swelling which does not extend over the suture line. It is usually present over one of the parietal bones. This swelling undergoes gradual absorption and usually disappears some weeks after birth. No active treatment is necessary but the mother should be reassured. Aspiration should not be performed, as there is always the danger of sepsis. The differentiating features between a cephalhaematoma and a caput are that the cephalhaematoma has a gradual onset, is limited to one bone, has heaped up edges and disappears slowly whereas a caput has not these features.

Cranial bones. The cranial bones may be fractured during delivery, especially when forceps are used, or when the head presses upon the sacral promontory during birth. The varieties of fractures are the depressed type which is usually spoonshaped (pond fracture), and the linear, stellate or comminuted fracture, when the parietal bones are most often involved. The fracture itself is of importance only if associated with intracranial injury.

Intracranial injuries

Very large cerebral haemorrhages are not compatible with life. The haemorrhages that may occur are either extradural, subdural, subarachnoid, intraventricular or intracerebral. They may be supra- or infratentorial depending on whether they are above or below the tentorium cerebelli. The infant having a cerebral injury usually has poor respiratory function with asphyxial attacks, and has a high-pitched cerebral cry. The pulse may be variable and the child does not suck well. If the haemorrhage is supratentorial, the anterior fontanelle is usually tense,

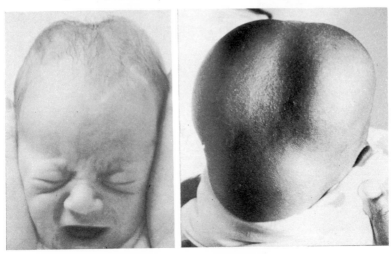

Fig. 5.20 Bilateral cephalhaematomata in a newborn infant.
Fig. 5.21 Another newborn infant with three cephalhaematomata (one over the occipital bone and the others over each parietal bone of the skull).

with poor pulsation. Convulsions may occur in any case of cerebral haemorrhage, and they may be bilateral or mixed in type. In these cases lumbar puncture will show blood-stained cerebrospinal fluid (the cerebrospinal fluid of the normal newborn child usually has a few red cells present). The Moro reflex is diminished or absent. The blood clotting abnormality of disseminated intravascular coagulation may be a factor in intracranial haemorrhage.

Treatment

The ideal treatment is the prevention of such happenings and this prevention is an obstetrical problem. The use of vitamin K_1 in proper dosage should be encouraged to aid blood clotting, but not in excess. Oxygen must be given and the child should be handled as gently as possible. Irritability, twitching and convulsions should be treated by sedation using a preparation such as chloral hydrate. In cases of subdural haematoma, treatment requires the removal of the blood by the procedure of subdural tapping.

Extracranial injuries

These may occur when labour has been difficult, especially in breech deliveries and forceps extractions, and include the following conditions:

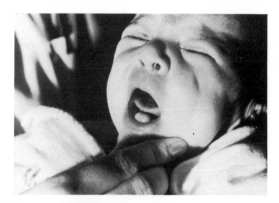

Fig. 5.22 Ranula (cyst under the tongue).

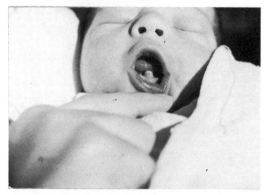

Fig. 5.23 Supernumerary tooth present at birth.

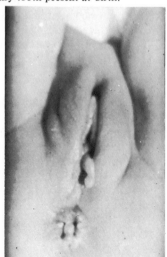

Fig. 5.24 Hymenal tag.

Spinal injuries. These injuries are very rare and are usually associated with breech deliveries and extension of the head. They are usually fatal.

Fractured clavicle. This injury is not uncommon and may be easily missed. Both vertex and breech deliveries are liable to the injury. It is of minor consequence and heals rapidly without special treatment.

Fractured humerus. This fracture may occur in a breech delivery with extended arms. The break is usually in the upper half of the humerus and heals very rapidly with much callus formation.

Fractured femur. This injury usually occurs when a leg is brought down during breech delivery; treatment requires suspension of the legs in a Gallow splint.

Nerve injuries. The facial nerve may be injured, especially in forceps deliveries where the blade causes pressure on the nerve (Fig. 5.25). The facial paralysis is easily diagnosed and this injury usually improves in a few weeks.

Brachial plexus injuries. The brachial plexus may be injured if stretched by wide separation of the neck from the shoulder or in bringing down an arm in delivery. The fifth and sixth cervical nerves may be affected producing the Erb-Duchenne paralysis (Figs 5.26 and 5.27). This paralysis causes the arm to hang at the side of the child in the so-called porter's tip position. The treatment requires abduction of the arm, flexion of the elbow and supination of the forearm in an appropriate splint or with pillows placed in the appropriate position, although some authorities allow free movement of the affected limb. These cases usually improve completely in about 12 weeks. The eighth cervical and the first thoracic nerves of the brachial plexus may also be injured,

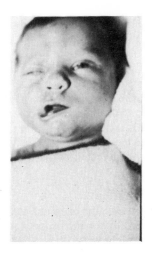

Fig. 5.25 Right facial palsy in a newborn child due to a difficult forceps delivery.

producing Klumpke's paralysis. With this type the forearm is in a position of supination with the hand in a claw position.

Visceral injuries. If the liver and spleen are ruptured, as may occur during a difficult delivery, the results are usually fatal. So it is too with suprarenal haemorrhage.

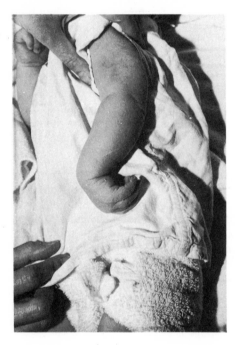

Fig. 5.26 Newborn infant with Erb-Duchenne paralysis showing the position of the paralysed limb.

Sternomastoid tumour. A haematoma may occur in the sheath of the sternomastoid muscle after certain deliveries, especially breech. A firm swelling develops about the size of a walnut; this swelling is hard and non-tender. In very rare cases torticollis may be a sequel, but with proper physiotherapy this serious complication should not occur. The mother should be instructed in the proper management in relation to maintaining mobility of the affected muscle.

Asphyxia and anoxia

This term implies that the foetus or infant has not a sufficient oxygen supply for its needs, especially for the proper functioning of the central nervous system. Anoxia might occur in the foetus. For proper oxygen carriage from mother to foetus the mother's blood must be healthy, the placenta and umbilical cord must function properly and the circulatory system of the foetus must be normal. On this basis toxaemia of pregnancy or other illness in the mother, depressant drugs, accidental haemorrhage, placental insufficiency, a knot of the umbilical cord and

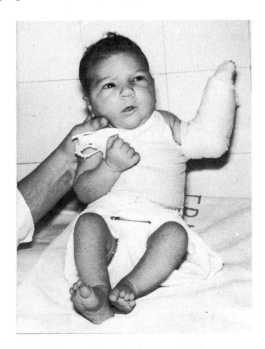

Fig. 5.27 The same infant as in Fig. 5.26 with the paralysed limb splinted in the appropriate position.

haemolysis of the baby's blood might produce anoxia of the foetus. Foetal anoxia and hypoxia is an important cause of foetal and neonatal (perinatal) death and methods of earlier detection are available to allow for improved control. These methods of detection of foetal anoxia giving rise to foetal distress include foetal monitoring of ECG with electronic equipment such as the cardiotocograph, and also the obstetric method of amnioscopy (for viewing the colour of the amniotic fluid) and also biochemical assessment of the foetus performed on blood specimens taken from the presenting part of the foetus usually the scalp. Other methods of assessing foetal wellbeing include the measurement of maternal urinary oestriol output.

After birth adequate oxygenation of the baby requires a properly functioning respiratory centre, clear air passages and normal lungs and cardiovascular system. Asphyxial states therefore might occur in prematurity, cerebral injuries or drug depression of the respiratory centre. The air passages might be obstructed with inhaled amniotic products or the hyaline membrane syndrome might occur. This syndrome usually affects the premature baby, the infant born to the diabetic mother or the post-Caesarean section infant. Abnormalities of the lungs or cardiovascular system, such as congenital heart disease, might produce a cyanotic state and acute respiratory distress may also be caused by a diaphragmatic hernia or by a pneumothorax.

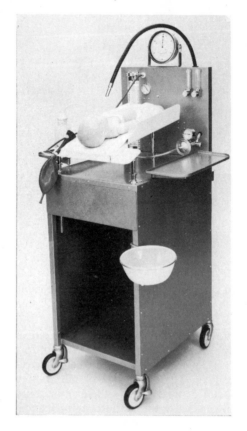

Fig. 5.28 Infant resuscitation trolley. (*By courtesy of Vickers Ltd.*)

Clinical signs

Asphyxia has a wide range of severity and clinical features include a variety of symptoms such as apnoea, irregularity of respiratory rhythm, sternal and intercostal retraction, expiratory grunting, cyanosis and circulatory collapse. Haemorrhagic states might also follow. A suitable method of assessing the condition of a newborn infant at birth is the Apgar rating; for this assessment, up to two marks are given for each of five features in relation to heart rate, respiratory function, reflex irritability, colour and muscle tone. An Apgar score of 10 is the ideal condition of the infant.

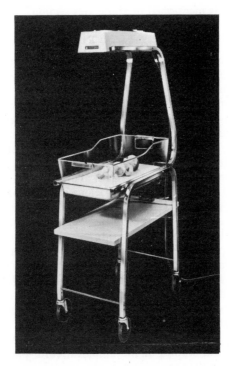

Fig. 5.29 Infant warmer.

The treatment of these conditions requires the usual general care of the child, including keeping the infant warm and using very gentle handling. The airways must be kept clear. Great gentleness must be exercised in this procedure and a rubber mucus extractor may be used; the child should be nursed with the head down.

It is important that assistance be given to establish respiration. Oxygen is the main requirement and the most effective treatment is intubation of the trachea followed by intermittent positive-pressure inflation of the lungs. Use has been made of stimulant drugs such as ethamivan (Vandid) and nikethamide administered sublingually, as they are absorbed by the mucous membrane of the mouth but they are of doubtful benefit. It is necessary to reiterate that the main requirement is oxygenation.

In cases of asphyxia of the newborn where the cause is depression of the respiratory centre by morphia or pethidine given to the mother before delivery, the drug nalorphine (Lethidrone) should be given.

Respiratory function must be maintained. The acute respiratory distress syndrome with hyaline membrane formation in the lungs requires the use of biochemical control, humidity, oxygen therapy and other measures as mentioned in a previous section.

INFECTION

The newborn infant has very little resistance to infection and has an open wound present at the umbilicus. Infection may develop antenatally, during the birth process, and postnatally.

Various antenatal infections may be acquired before birth and these include syphilis, rarely malaria, various virus infections and the protozoal infection with *Toxoplasma gondii* producing congenital toxoplasmosis. During birth the child may contract a gonorrhoeal infection of the eyes (gonococcal ophthalmia) and also a monilial infection of the mouth (thrush) from the mother. In the post-natal period the child may be infected by various bacterial organisms such as staphylococci, streptococci, *Escherichia coli* and other bacteria, and also by viruses and the fungus *Monilia albicans* (*Candida albicans*). It is recognised that newborn infants are susceptible to many bacteria which are less pathogenic to the older age-group; this applies particularly to the Gram-negative coliform organisms. Soon after birth newborn infants may become colonised with a bacterial flora affecting the skin, the upper respiratory and the alimentary tracts. Antenatal infections might occur where the mother has premature rupture of membranes, although this is not a necessary factor in ascending infection of the foetus. In these cases it is recommended that rapid, frozen-section histological studies of the umbilical cord, placenta and membranes be undertaken to assist in the proper assessment of these infants; these studies may support antenatal infection by finding evidence of inflammatory reaction in the cord, placenta and membranes. Newborn infants traumatised by a difficult delivery are particularly likely to be affected by Gram-negative bacterial infection.

Septicaemia

This condition may go unrecognised as there may not be an obvious primary focus and there may also not be any of the signs of septicaemia as found in an older patient. The symptoms may be rapid dehydration, vomiting, diarrhoea or haemorrhages. There may not be any pyrexia but these infants are usually extremely ill. A blood culture may bring to light the responsible organism. Treatment should be an attack on the causative organism with antibiotic therapy, together with general supportive treatment.

Skin infections

The skin of a newborn baby is delicate and may be easily injured by excessive zeal in cleaning. The infections, often staphylococcal, may affect the skin as the condition of pemphigus neonatorum or bullous impetigo. The infection can be controlled by the use of antibiotics, and cases that occur in a nursery should also be immediately isolated and

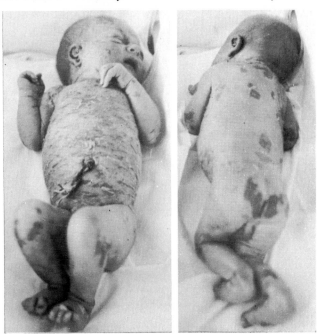

Fig. 5.30 A newborn infant with congenital ichthyosiform erythroderma which resembled Ritter's disease.
Fig. 5.31 The back of the same child as in previous figure.

barrier nursed, to prevent spread. The possible source of the infection should be looked for in the attendants of the nursery. In some cases exfoliation takes place, producing the condition known as Ritter's disease (Figs 5.30 and 5.31). This disease responds fairly well to antibiotic therapy. The skin may also be affected by a folliculitis and impetigo, and nail infections (paronychiae) may also occur.

Eye infections

Gonorrhoeal ophthalmia may be produced by infection during the birth process as mentioned previously; this disease has become uncommon with improving antenatal services which detect gonococcal infection of the mother during pregnancy. The disease responds well to antimicrobial agents such as penicillin. The eyelids may also be affected by a staphylococcal blepharitis. A trachoma-inclusion conjunctivitis agent (TRIC) has been identified as a possible cause of conjunctival infection in the newborn.

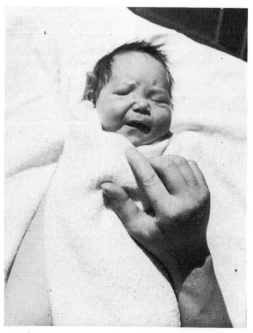

Fig. 5.32 Newborn infant with a right dacryocystitis (inflammatory lesion of the lachrymal sac).

Umbilical infections (omphalitis)

The umbilicus of a newborn infant is an open wound and may be infected by staphylococcal, streptococcal, pneumococcal, diphtheritic, gonococcal and tetanus organisms. In the pus-coccal infections there is usually a purulent discharge at the base of the umbilical stump. This separates slowly and bleeding may occur. The condition may become more severe, and the infection may spread up the umbilical vessels, producing abscesses in the liver with jaundice and septicaemia. A granuloma may form later at the infected umbilicus, and this may give rise to a chronic discharge. This granulomatous polyp can be treated with the application of a silver nitrate stick. Tetanus of the newborn is very rare but does occasionally occur. The child is very sensitive to any stimulus and there is difficulty in sucking; convulsions usually follow, and the condition has a very high mortality. Active immunisation with tetanus toxoid during pregnancy may be useful in preventing neonatal tetanus in areas where this disease occurs.

Alimentary tract infections

The mouth of the newborn infant is delicate and the mucosa may be easily traumatised. The mouth may be infected with thrush, which is due to a fungus, *Monilia albicans.* In this infection there are small, whitish patches covering the mucosa of the tongue, palate, cheek and lips. The treatment requires the use of nystatin. Diarrhoea in the newborn may occur. This is usually a very serious disease and may spread rapidly amongst other infants in a nursery. The cause is unknown, but a virus is being incriminated as the cause of this condition. The infant has loose, frequent stools and becomes rapidly dehydrated and toxic. Therapy requires the use of intravenous fluids with the possible addition of an antibiotic; the rapid isolation of these cases is necessary to prevent spread in a nursery.

Respiratory tract infections

During the birth process the infant may inhale infected liquor amnii producing a pneumonia. After birth, infants who have atelectasis may develop pneumonia with its serious consequences.

Meningeal infections

Meningitis may occur in the neonatal period. The commonest organism to produce this in this age-group is the *Escherichia coli*, although other organisms such as the meningococcus, pneumococcus or *Listeria monocytogenes* might also produce the same infection. The infant in this age-group often has no obvious signs of meningeal irritation and the condition may be difficult to diagnose. Lumbar puncture is essential in the diagnosis of this disease.

Urinary tract infection

This may occur in the neonate due to infection by *Escherichia coli.*

Ear infections

Ear infection may follow a pharyngitis and may be associated with the baby being fed with the head in a low position.

Bone infections

Osteomyelitis may occur in the newborn period and any bone such as the humerus, femur, tibia or ulna may be affected. This disease responds quite well to early therapy with penicillin or other appropriate antibiotic.

Coxsackie B virus infection

This virus, of which there are six strains, is known to cause Born-holm's disease (epidemic pleurodynia) in adults and children; this disease is a self-limited condition with pyrexia, constitutional disturbance and severe pain in the chest and abdomen. In the newborn infant, however, infection with the Coxsackie B virus may be highly dangerous as it may cause a neonatal myocarditis (an inflammatory lesion of the heart muscle) and encephalitis. The symptomatology of this neonatal Coxsackie B myocarditis includes listlessness, feeding difficulty, pyrexia, tachycardia, respiratory distress, cyanosis and cardiac failure; symptomatic treatment should be given but the disease has a high mortality and therefore should be prevented if possible.

The herpes simplex virus might also infect the newborn infant; this is fortunately rare as this type of infection in this age-group is extremely dangerous. Cytomegalovirus infection is another serious condition which may be transmitted antenatally from the mother via the placenta. This disease may produce jaundice, hepatosplenomegaly (enlarged liver and spleen), petechial haemorrhages and microcephaly with calcifications in the brain and has a high mortality.

HAEMORRHAGIC CONDITIONS

The blood vessels in the newborn child are delicate, especially in the premature infant, and this makes them more liable to haemorrhage; in

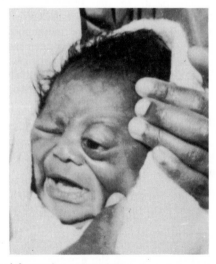

Fig. 5.33 Proptosis of the left eye of a newborn infant due to haemorrhagic disease of the newborn (haemorrhage behind the eyeball). The condition regressed to complete normality. (*By courtesy from Kessel & Glynn Williams: 'South African Medical Journal'*.)

addition, birth trauma and anoxia increase the liability to haemorrhage. Overlying these causes, the newborn child has a low plasma prothrombin with an increased clotting time. These facts may make haemorrhage occur in this age-group. Neonatal haemorrhage, therefore, may be due to birth trauma, asphyxial states, infections such as septicaemia and syphilis, haemorrhagic disease of the newborn (hypoprothrombinaemia), umbilical haemorrhage and the very rare conditions such as haemophilia and thrombocytopenia (reduced platelets).

Haemorrhagic disease of the newborn

This condition affects less than one in 500 births, and is associated with the low plasma prothrombin in the neonate. The bleeding usually occurs on the second to fifth day and affects most commonly the bowel (melaena neonatorum) producing black, tarry stools. Haemorrhage from the umbilicus occurs next in frequency, and haematemesis, skin bleeding or haemorrhage from the nose or urinary tract might also occur. The bleeding may be severe and give rise to a very shocked baby, the severity depending upon the amount of blood lost. In order to increase the prothrombin of the blood, vitamin K_1 is essential, and this may be given to the mother from 4 to 12 hours before the child is born, or to the baby as treatment for the condition in a dosage of 2·5 mg, by intramuscular injection of the aqueous solution. This may be repeated in six hours. If the blood loss has been large a blood transfusion is essential. It should be stressed that newborn infants stand blood loss badly and it must be remembered in this regard that the total blood volume of infants is only approximately 85 ml per kg bodyweight.

Umbilical haemorrhage

Bleeding from the umbilicus may occur if the ligature tying the cord has slipped or has cut through. This usually occurs on the first day of life. The use of an elastic band instead of the usual ligature may be useful in better control of umbilical haemorrhage. From the second to the fifth day the bleeding is usually due to haemorrhagic disease of the newborn. Infection and congenital syphilis might also produce haemorrhage. After the first week, an umbilical granuloma or polyp may start bleeding. These umbilical granulomata may respond to the application of silver nitrate or may require surgical excision; it is necessary in these cases of possible granulomatous lesions to exclude the possibility of them being associated with a Meckel's diverticulum (vitello-intestinal duct) or urachal remnant which would require more extensive surgery.

NEONATAL JAUNDICE

Icterus, or jaundice, is a common condition in the newborn child. It is a symptom and describes the yellow staining of the skin and mucous membranes by the bile pigment bilirubin. It may be due to various causes:

1. 'Physiological'
2. Haemolytic disease of the newborn (erythroblastosis foetalis): Rh incompatibility; ABO incompatibility
3. Infections—septicaemia, syphilis, sepsis
4. Congenital obliteration of the bile ducts
5. Inspissated bile syndrome
6. Hepatitis (viral, toxoplasmosis)
7. Rarer causes, such as hereditary spherocytosis (acholuric jaundice), galactosaemia, cretinism (hypothyroidism), absorbing haematoma, 'breast milk jaundice' etc.

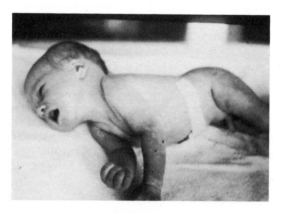

Fig. 5.34 Kernicterus in severely jaundiced newborn infant.

There is widening interest in the whole field of neonatology including that of neonatal jaundice. The basis of this interest has been the recognition that severe jaundice (hyperbilirubinaemia) in the immediate neonatal period subjects the infant to the grave danger of developing brain damage in the form of kernicterus or bilirubin encephalopathy. Kernicterus is the name given to the yellow staining of brain cells particularly of the corpus striatum and is a condition which only affects the brain of the infant in the immediate newborn period. This kernicterus complication of the heavily jaundiced neonate may be rapidly fatal or be responsible for producing a handicapped child with such severe sequelae as cerebral palsy with or without athetosis, mental subnormality or deafness. In view of this danger it is now standard practice to be watchful in the management of jaundice in the newborn. The further extension of investigation into aspects of kernicterus complicating neonatal hyperbilirubinaemia has provided information in regard to the differences between unconjugated and conjugated bilirubin circulating in the serum. Bilirubin has its origin as one of the breakdown products of haemoglobin by the reticulo-

TABLE 1

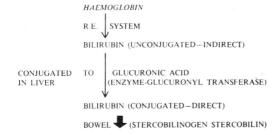

JAUNDICE (ICTERUS)—
RAISED BLOOD BILIRUBIN STAINING TISSUES YELLOW

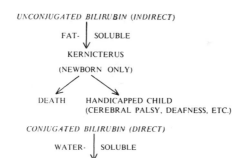

TYPES OF JAUNDICE

1. HAEMOLYTIC (EXCESS RED BLOOD CELL DESTRUCTION)
2. OBSTRUCTIVE (OBSTRUCTION TO BILE OUTFLOW)
3. HEPATIC (LIVER CELL DISEASE)

endothelial (R.E.) system; this bilirubin (unconjugated or indirect-reading) circulates in the blood and is conjugated to glucuronic acid in the liver with the aid of the enzyme glucuronyl transferase to form conjugated or direct-reading bilirubin; this then passes into the biliary system to take its place in the formation of bile. It is now recognised that unconjugated bilirubin (indirect reading) is responsible for producing kernicterus. It is also recognised that any marked rise of this bilirubin from whatever cause in the immediate neonatal period might be complicated by kernicterus. The recognition of the kernicteric danger to the heavily jaundiced newborn infant makes it imperative that, notwithstanding the particular cause of the jaundice, active steps be taken to keep the circulating serum unconjugated bilirubin level within reasonable limits. These active steps, at the present time, require the use of adequate exchange transfusion to reduce the serum bilirubin to safe limits; this may require repeated exchange transfusions to safeguard the infant. Other therapeutic approaches are also available and these include phototherapy by exposing these infants to blue light to reduce the bilirubin levels (Fig. 5.35), and also the administration of phenobarbitone which appears to increase the hepatic glucuronyl transferase enzyme activity for the conjugation of bilirubin. This form of treatment using phenobarbitone may be more effective if given to

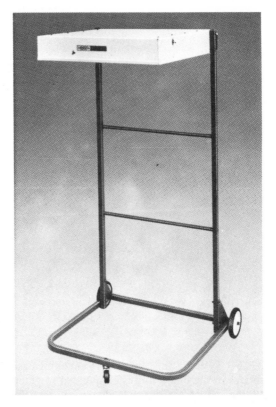

Fig. 5.35 Phototherapy unit for the treatment of neonatal jaundice to lower serum bilirubin levels.

the pregnant mother in the last week or two of pregnancy in addition to the infant after birth and this combined treatment of both mother and child appears to give a better result than treatment of the newborn alone.

'Physiological' jaundice

This condition occurs in a high proportion of normal newborn infants, and the premature baby has an increased predisposition to it. The jaundice usually appears on the third day and disappears by the tenth to the fourteenth day. There are no symptoms except occasional lethargy and difficulty in feeding. The cause is related to the infant's high red blood cell count at birth and their rapid breakdown giving rise to an excess of bile pigment. The liver is functionally immature and cannot deal with this excess pigment, which therefore accumulates in the blood and produces jaundice.

It appears that overdosage with synthetic vitamin K may act as an oxidising agent producing haemolysis and be responsible for causing newborn infants to become jaundiced; this has been the reason for reducing the dosage of this vitamin administered to the newborn infant, where indicated. Vitamin K_1 (Konakion) is usually prescribed as a safer preparation in a dose of 1 mg for the full-term infant and 0·5 mg for the premature and low birth weight infants for prophylactic use in preventing haemorrhagic disease in certain cases. As mentioned elsewhere in this book other drugs such as the sulphonamides (e.g. sulphafurazole, Gantrisin) may also produce jaundice, sometimes complicated by kernicterus in the newborn infant, particularly when premature. Sulphonamides may also be harmful to the newborn infant if administered to the pregnant mother in late pregnancy; the action of this drug in producing jaundice is that it competes with bilirubin for sites of attachment on albumen with a subsequent rise in circulating bilirubin. Another preparation having a similar effect but for a different reason is the antibiotic novobiocin which appears to interfere with the excretion process of bilirubin through the liver.

Haemolytic disease of the newborn (erythroblastosis foetalis—icterus gravis neonatorum)

Rh incompatibility. This disease occurs because of Rh incompatibility between mother and child. Where the blood of the mother is Rh negative, that of the father and of the foetus *in utero* Rh positive, this may allow her sensitisation to the Rh-positive cells of the infant. Rh-positive foetal red blood cells may cross the placenta back to the mother and so sensitise her; the mother's next contact with an Rh-positive foetus (i.e. another Rh-positive pregnancy) may stimulate her to produce Rh antibodies which would pass back through the placenta to the foetus and affect its red blood cells by destroying them by the process of haemolysis. This disease may present itself clinically as hydrops foetalis, icterus gravis neonatorum or haemolytic anaemia of the newborn. Cases of hydrops foetalis are usually stillborn. Icterus gravis occurs as jaundice from birth or very soon afterwards, becoming rapidly more intense. There is an associated anaemia with the child's blood count and haemoglobin dropping rapidly. There are many nucleated red cells in the baby's circulation and the serum bilirubin content often rises to high levels. The Coombs test performed on umbilical cord blood is positive in these cases, which indicates that the baby's red blood cells have been sensitised to Rh antibodies and that the child is suffering from erythroblastosis foetalis. This disease does not usually affect the first child of a pregnancy where the mother is Rh negative, the father Rh positive and the baby Rh positive, unless the mother has been previously sensitised to the Rh factor by having had a transfusion of Rh-positive blood (Fig. 5.36). The second child of such a couple may be affected, possibly mildly, and any subsequent

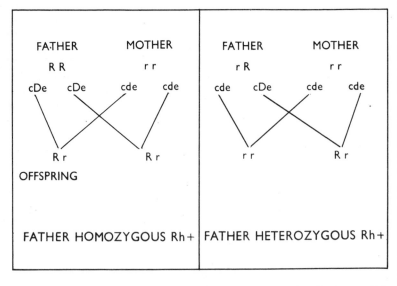

Fig. 5.36 Diagram illustrating the genetic transmission of the Rh factor. (RR indicates homozygous Rh-positive individuals, Rr heterozygous Rh-positive and rr Rh-negative individuals.)

children are usually more severely affected. One of the most serious complications of this disease is kernicterus, where the nerve cells of the basal ganglia of the brain are stained yellow. This complication develops on the second or third day, when the child may twitch, become stiff, have a high-pitched cerebral cry, and may develop convulsions. If such a child survives, he may later develop spasticity, mental retardation, deafness or cerebral palsy.

Treatment

The best treatment is exchange transfusion with Rh negative group O blood (not the mother's) or preferably the same group as the baby. The amount of blood usually used in this exchange transfusion is about 160 to 220 ml per kg bodyweight (80 to 100 ml/lb), and the results have been very good. In some cases, repeat exchange transfusions may be necessary if the child becomes more jaundiced. The breast milk of the mother contains Rh antibodies, but this is not absorbed by the child after the second day of life and therefore this condition is not a contraindication to breast feeding. A routine check on the serum bilirubin level and the haemoglobin is necessary after the exchange transfusion. In the prediction of severity of the disease in the foetus, use is being made of the examination of liquor amnii obtained by amniocentesis. For very severe affection of the foetus Liley in New Zealand has described the method of treatment of intrauterine intraperitoneal transfusion of the foetus. A method is available to prevent Rh-negative women becoming sensitised by their Rh-positive foetuses. This protection against Rh sensitisation is done by injecting these mothers with human immunoglobulin containing the Rh (anti-D) antibody shortly after delivery, thereby destroying foetal Rh-positive red cells circulating in the mother's circulation. This method is very successful in preventing this type of haemolytic disease of the newborn. Before this method of prevention was available about 10 to 20 per cent of Rh-negative mothers with Rh-positive fathers produced babies with haemolytic disease of the newborn.

ABO incompatibility. This condition is similar to erythroblastosis foetalis except that the incompatibility is not due to the Rh factor but to the ABO groups (Fig. 5.37). In these cases the Coombs test is usually negative and the disease may affect the first child. The mother's blood group is usually O and the baby group A (or B), the father being also group A (or B). It should be stressed, however, that only very few babies born of this combination of blood groups are affected by this disease. The treatment for severe cases of ABO incompatibility with jaundice is also exchange transfusion.

Infections

Any severe septic condition in the child, such as septicaemia or the complications of umbilical infection, may produce jaundice. The treatment will be relative to the cause.

Congenital syphilis. This condition might also affect the liver and be accompanied by jaundice. There are usually other signs of the disease and the jaundice is of bad prognostic significance.

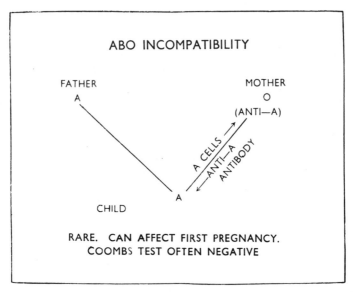

Fig. 5.37 Diagram illustrating the manner in which ABO incompatibility operates to produce this type of jaundice in the newborn.

Atresia of the bile ducts

In this condition there is abnormality of the bile channels, which might be either in the liver (intrahepatic) or outside the liver (extra-hepatic). This abnormality obstructs the flow of bile and produces an obstructive jaundice. The infant usually becomes jaundiced towards the end of the first week and this becomes progressively worse. The stools are pale, and the urine dark with bile pigments. The treatment is surgical and will only be successful if the obstruction is extrahepatic, when an anastomotic operation may be performed. The prognosis is usually poor, although these infants may survive many months and even years. There may be great difficulty in differentiating this condition from neonatal hepatitis and the condition may possibly be a sequel to intrauterine hepatitis. A useful test is the ^{131}I rose bengal excretion test in which the faecal excretion of the radioisotope is measured in the 72 hours after intravenous injection (less than 8 per cent indicates lack of bile flow). Other tests which may be useful to distinguish neonatal hepatitis from atresia of the bile ducts are the serum levels of alpha-fetoprotein and of lipoprotein. A most useful investigation in the differential diagnosis of these conditions is cholangiography and also percutaneous liver biopsy.

Neonatal hepatitis

This disease may occur in the newborn infant due to many different causes. Viral infection may occur from the mother antenatally via the placenta. The clinical jaundice may occur at any time and abnormality of liver function tests are helpful in the diagnosis. Deficiency of alpha-1-antitrypsin has been shown to be an important factor in liver disease. This substance is a glycoprotein synthesised in the liver and deficiency may occur as a genetically determined condition (normal concentration in the serum is 200 mg per 100 ml); in early adult life this deficiency may be associated with emphysema.

Inspissated bile syndrome

In this condition there is obstruction to the bile ducts by inspissated thickened bile. It is seen rarely in cases of haemolytic disease of the newborn with hyperbilirubinaemia. This condition must be differentiated from atresia of the bile ducts.

Some rarer causes

There is the familial disease of hereditary spherocytosis which may be transmitted as a dominant trait where an infant may be affected if one of the parents has the condition. It is due to an abnormality of the red cells with increased destruction of these by the spleen. This disease usually presents with symptoms at a later age and only rarely presents with jaundice in the neonatal period.

There are other extremely rare causes of jaundice in the newborn, such as galactosaemia and cretinism (hypothyroidism). This latter condition appears to delay maturation of the conjugating system; these diseases are considered elsewhere in this book. It is necessary to stress the importance of early diagnosis in these cases to obtain the best response to early treatment.

Any large haemorrhage such as a cephalhaematoma, in its absorption, may also produce jaundice in the infant.

A rare condition known as 'breast milk jaundice' is recognised as a possible cause of jaundice in the immediate neonatal period; this is due to the presence of a steroid substance in breast milk (pregnane-3 α, 20 β-diol) which depresses enzyme activity and delays the proper conjugation of bilirubin. Jaundice may also be found rarely in infants with pyloric stenosis.

Another very rare cause is the Crigler-Najjar syndrome (familial non-haemolytic jaundice with kernicterus), which is due to a deficiency of the enzyme glucuronyl transferase; this appears to be a recessive disease. Another syndrome, Gilbert's disease, also has jaundice as a feature but the onset is usually at puberty; it appears to affect males only and kernicterus does not occur.

MISCELLANEOUS CONDITIONS

Anaemia

Anaemic conditions in the newborn occur most readily in the preterm low birth weight infant or following any infection. It is part of the picture of haemolytic disease of the newborn and may also follow haemorrhagic disease of the newborn. On rare occasions an infant may be born pale with severe anaemia due to a bleed into the mother's circulation *in utero* via the placenta (foetomaternal transplacental haemorrhage). In this condition confirmation of the presence of large numbers of foetal red cells in the maternal circulation may be found using the Kleihauer technique. A rather similar situation may be seen in one of monozygotic twins with a conjoined placental circulation in which one twin may bleed into the other. In this case one is found to be pale and anaemic and the other plethoric with a high red blood cell count and high haemoglobin. A similar foetal haemorrhage might follow incision through the placenta in patients undergoing a lower segment Caesarean section operation for an anterior placenta praevia. In those infants with severe anaemia, urgent blood transfusion is necessary.

Mastitis neonatorum (Fig. 5.38)

Swelling of the breasts may occur in either sex a few days after birth. The breasts become quite tense and may secrete a watery colostrum-like fluid. The condition is due to hormonal carry-over from the mother and

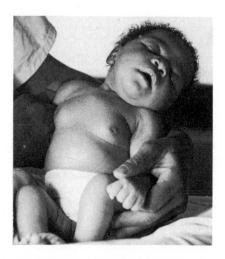

Fig. 5.38 A newborn infant with bilateral enlargement of the breasts—the condition of mastitis neonatorum.

always clears up, therefore no treatment is necessary. The swellings should not be squeezed or otherwise interfered with as this may introduce infection leading to the development of a true mastitis with suppuration. The hormonal carry-over may also produce a mucoid vaginal discharge and minor vaginal bleeding; this is of no consequence and has been called 'menstruation of the newborn'.

Inanition or dehydration fever

Some newborn infants develop a high temperature a few days after birth. This is usually associated with a low fluid intake and loss of weight. There may be some lethargy but there is no evidence of infection. These infants respond very well to giving adequate fluids by mouth.

Neonatal cold injury

It is clear that the newborn infant may be harmed by cold; the earliest symptoms are lethargy and refusing feeds followed by the development of oedema. It is interesting to note that a similar problem of hypothermia can affect the older age groups in the geriatric field of medicine. The infant feels cold and may develop a pinkish appearance of the face and a nasal discharge. Temperatures as low as 26·7°C (80°F) have been recorded in this syndrome and the condition is highly dangerous. Hypoglycaemia (low blood glucose level) may be an associated condition and requires that glucose feeds be given; these patients need to be warmed *gradually* and should be given an antibiotic to cover infection. There is a high risk of pulmonary haemorrhage complicating the clinical picture and this is often fatal. The main cause of this hypothermic syndrome developing appears to be a low surrounding environmental temperature and this should be guarded against. A low-reading thermometer is a necessary item of equipment in the care of young infants both full term and preterm.

Offspring of diabetic mothers

There is a higher foetal and neonatal death rate in the offspring of diabetic mothers than in the normal population but nevertheless with the proper care and control of these patients many such babies survive; these do not themselves become diabetic. These infants are usually large and overweight even when premature. They should be managed in the same way as low birth weight and premature infants notwithstanding their weight and size. If these infants are born by Caesarean section, as they frequently are, it should be routine practice to aspirate their stomach contents soon after birth to prevent regurgitation and possible inhalation; this emptying of the stomach after birth should be a routine practice in all infants born by Caesarean section. Infants born of diabetic mothers are liable to develop the respiratory distress syndrome together with its grave dangers. These babies must be carefully assessed in relation to the possible development of hypoglycaemia (low blood glucose) and regular blood glucose levels must be done and the condition treated if the levels fall. For rapid estimation of blood glucose levels a glucose oxidase test paper (Dextrostix) can be used.

Neonatal surgery

There has been great development in the surgery of the newborn infant particularly in relation to congenital abnormalities. Advances in the technique of anaesthesia in the newborn period and in pre- and postoperative management have led to successful surgery in this age-group. Some of these abnormalities are discussed in other sections and include such conditions as oesophageal atresia with a tracheo-oesophageal fistula, duodenal atresia and imperforate anus. It is an accepted fact that newborn infants, under suitable conditions, respond well to surgery. Modern neonatal surgery requires a highly specialised medical and surgical team in addition to expert nursing care. Certain essential features are necessary in the proper pre- and postoperative management. Fluid therapy must be well controlled in regard to content and quantity in the first week after birth. The fluid requirements of the newborn child in the first week are less than the older infant, and this point cannot be sufficiently stressed. Early diagnosis is essential in these problems requiring neonatal surgery. Furthermore, it is necessary that infection be prevented in this vulnerable age-group.

Chromosomes

The study of chromosomes in man has been rapidly expanded. It is now recognised that the human somatic cell has 46 chromosomes which includes 22 pairs of autosomal chromosomes and the paired sex chromosomes (XX in the female and XY in the male). The sex germ cell (the ovum in the female and sperm in the male) have half the total number. Many chromosomal aberrations have been recognised; furthermore, the sex chromatin pattern of buccal mucosal cells or skin biopsy cells suitably stained show abnormality in the individuals with sex chromosome aberration. In normal females a chromatin body or mass (Barr body) is present in the nucleus of the cell as examined in a suitably stained buccal mucosal smear or skin biopsy specimen and also present as a drumstick-shaped appendage attached to the nucleus of a polymorphonuclear leucocyte in a peripheral blood film suitably stained. This nuclear sex chromatin body is not present in the normal male. The sex chromosomal aberrations include the rare Turner's syndrome in a female (Figs 5.39 and 5.40); in this condition the patient has ovarian dysgenesis (amenorrhoea due to abnormal ovarian function), webbing

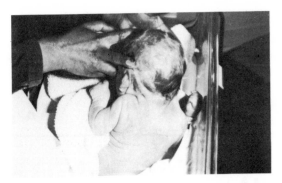

Fig. 5.39 Newborn infant showing webbing of the skin of the neck in the Bonnevie-Ullrich syndrome (Turner's syndrome). This syndrome has an abnormality of the sex chromosomes with the XO pattern.

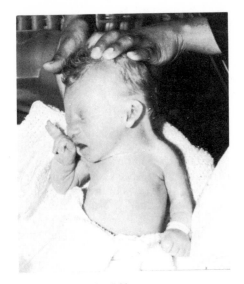

Fig. 5.40 The same infant as in Fig. 5.39.

of the skin of the neck, a low neck hair-line, increased angulation of the elbow joints (cubitus valgus), a broad chest with widely spaced nipples ('shield chest') and shortened height. These patients have been demonstrated as having 45 chromosomes with the sex chromosome XO pattern; they also frequently have a coarctation of the aorta present and show the male chromatin pattern of cell (chromatin negative). A similar condition known as the Bonnevie-Ullrich syndrome often has oedema of the feet present in the newborn period. Klinefelter's syndrome (Fig. 5.41) is another example of a sex chromosomal aberration in the male where there are a total of 47 chromosomes with a XXY

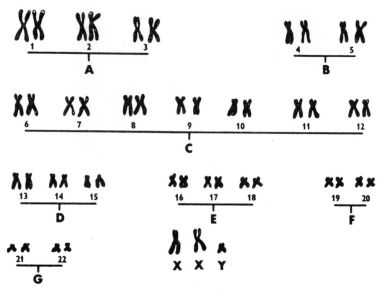

Fig. 5.41 Chromosomal pattern in Klinefelter's syndrome showing XXY. (*By courtesy from Emery: 'Elements of Medical Genetics'. Churchill Livingstone, Edinburgh.*)

pattern of sex chromosomes; these patients are usually mentally retarded, have testicular atrophy, enlarged breasts and a female sex chromatin pattern of cell (chromatin positive). Many other types of chromosomal aberrations have been described. An XXX female (triplo-X) with two chromatin bodies in the buccal mucosal cell or skin biopsy specimen has been described and also tetra-X (XXXX), triplo-X,Y (XXXY) and other varieties. These variations with additional X chromosomes have more than one chromatin body in the nucleus. A male individual with a sex chromosome pattern of XYY has also been described where interest lies in the possible association of these individuals with antisocial conduct, although this view is not generally accepted. A reliable technique for detecting the Y chromosome is the fluorescent staining of suitable cells. Patients with Down's syndrome (mongolism) have been demonstrated to have 47 chromosomes caused by a triplication (trisomy) of a small chromosome (no. 21, or trisomy G) (Fig. 5.42); variants of this mongol type have also been recorded, such as the translocation type which is much less common than the trisomy. In the translocation type, the parents' chromosomes may be normal in which case the risk of a recurrence of Down's syndrome in a future pregnancy is low as it is with trisomy 21, but if one parent (especially the mother) or both show chromosomal abnormality, the risk of recurrence in future pregnancies is high. Other autosomal chromosome trisomy abnormalities include Patau's syndrome with trisomy 13

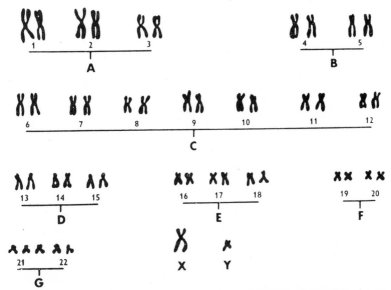

Fig. 5.42 Chromosomal pattern in Down's syndrome (mongolism) showing trisomy 21 (trisomy G). (*By courtesy from Emery: 'Elements of Medical Genetics'. Churchill Livingstone, Edinburgh.*)

(trisomy D) and Edward's syndrome of trisomy 18 (trisomy E). They have additional chromosomes with a total of 47 as is found in trisomy 21 (Down's syndrome, mongolism). They have multiple abnormalities and are usually fatal in the early months. Trisomy D (13) usually has severe cleft palate and lip with microphthalmia and microcephaly, and trisomy E (18) have overriding fingers (usually second over third), shortened or dorsiflexed big toe, 'rocker bottom' appearance of the feet, low-set ears with typical facies and other abnormalities.

A rare condition associated with a chromosomal abnormality (of autosomal chromosome 5) is the 'crying cat' syndrome (*le cri du chat* syndrome); in this condition there is microcephaly, micrognathos (hypoplastic mandible), epicanthic folds, hypertelorism, failure to thrive, mental retardation and a peculiar 'cat-like' cry due to a small larynx.

In relation to the prevention of certain congenital disorders, methods are being developed for determining these abnormalities in the foetus. These methods for prenatal diagnosis require the examination of foetal cells obtained by amniocentesis during pregnancy. The foetal amniotic cells may be examined and cultured for the study of the chromosomes (the karyotype of the individual). Congenital abnormalities with chromosomal aberrations such as Down's syndrome (mongolism) may be determined by this method and such pregnancies may be terminated. The sex determination of the foetus if male in a mother who is a carrier of an X-linked hereditary disease such as haemophilia or muscular dystrophy may also be important in prevention. Enzyme assays may also be done on material obtained by amniocentesis to detect deficiencies of enzymes in certain conditions such as Tay-Sachs disease (amaurotic family idiocy). Other techniques for the prenatal diagnosis

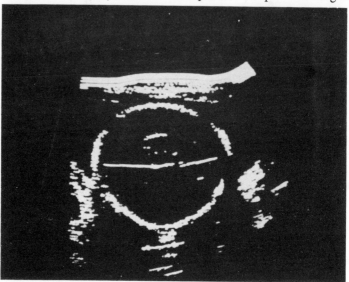

Fig. 5.43A Ultrasonic picture of a normal 30 weeks gestation pregnancy showing a normal biparietal diameter where the measurement is 8·1 cm. (Transverse scan.)

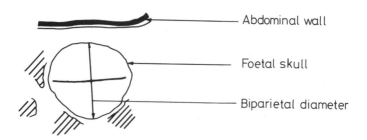

Fig. 5.43B Line drawing and interpretation of Fig. 5.43A.

of such conditions as meningomyelocele and encephalocele are being developed and these methods include the estimation of concentration of alpha-fetoprotein in the amniotic fluid, foetoscopy and ultrasonography (Figs 5.43 to 5.47).

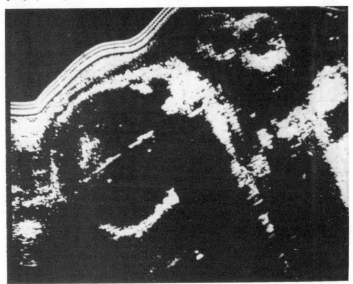

Fig. 5.44A Ultrasonic picture showing the foetal head in a 36-week pregnancy. (Longitudinal scan.)

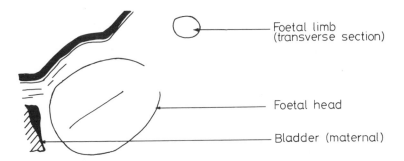

Fig. 5.44B Line drawing and interpretation of Fig. 5.44A.

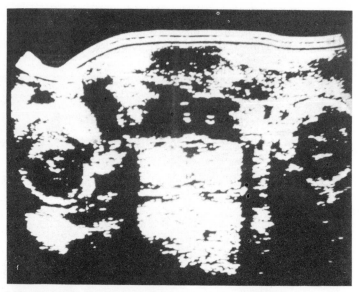

Fig. 5.45A Ultrasonic picture of a twin pregnancy showing the two heads and also the placental positions.

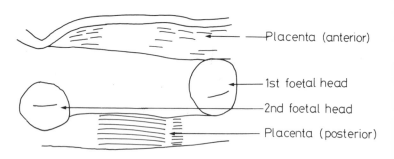

Fig. 5.45B Line drawing and interpretation of Fig. 5.45A.

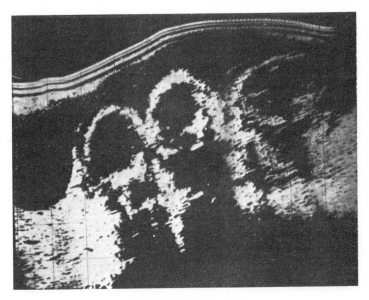

Fig. 5.46A Another ultrasonic picture of a twin pregnancy.

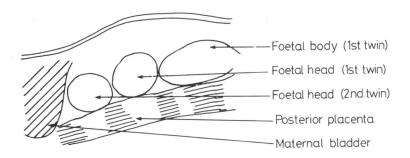

Fig. 5.46B Line drawing and interpretation of Fig. 5.46A.

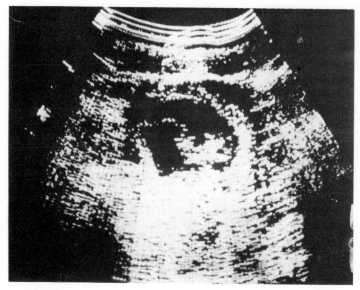

Fig. 5.47A Ultrasonic picture showing a 10-week pregnancy illustrating the foetus and possibly the umbilical cord.

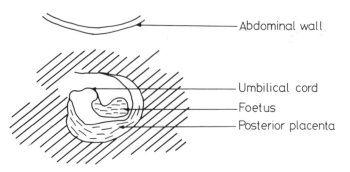

Fig. 5.47B Line drawing and interpretation of Fig. 5.47A.

6. Disorders of the Alimentary System

The gums and mucous membrane of the mouth may be involved in an inflammatory process. Gingivitis or inflammation of the gums is usually associated with bad teeth, and its prevention by good oral care should be the aim. Inflammation of the mucosa of the mouth (stomatitis) occurs in various forms due to different causes.

1. *Catarrhal stomatitis.* This is a mild affection where the mucosa is congested; it may be found in undernourished cases and may accompany measles. Measles itself is always associated with Koplik's spots. The treatment should aim at cleaning the mouth with a mild antiseptic.

2. *Aphthous stomatitis.* This is found in young children. Small raised whitish patches occur on the mucosa of the mouth; these patches drop off leaving shallow ulcers which are extremely painful. The condition may become more severe and lead to ulcerative stomatitis.

3. *Ulcerative stomatitis.* In this condition there are many shallow ulcers and in severe cases the gums may bleed. The breath is offensive and the mouth is tender. There may be general constitutional symptoms such as pyrexia and loss of appetite. It has been shown that this condition is caused by the virus of herpes simplex (*Herpesvirus hominis*); there may be secondary infection with the Vincent's organism producing Vincent's angina. The treatment, apart from general therapy, requires good oral hygiene. 5-iodo-2-Deoxyuridine (idoxuridine, IDU) is a preparation active against the virus of herpes simplex and is useful in the treatment of herpetic lesions of the cornea and may also be useful as a local application in the treatment of ulcerative stomatitis due to herpes virus.

4. *Gangrenous stomatitis.* This condition, also known as cancrum oris or noma, is fortunately extremely rare at the present time. It used to occur in very weakened children as a complication of infectious fevers. A deep gangrenous ulceration of the cheek occurs with necrosis of tissue and extreme toxaemia.

5. *Thrush.* This condition is due to a fungal infection of the mucosa of the mouth by *Monilia albicans* (*Candida albicans*). Young infants may be affected by contact with infected utensils when feeding. This condition has been discussed in the section on the newborn. It may spread down the oesophagus producing the serious disease of oesophagitis. In this condition the infant may vomit bloodstained material and

may inhale feed due to an inco-ordination of swallowing; for this serious disease with dissemination a useful therapeutic agent is ampho-tericin B (Fungizone—for infusion) by systemic administration. This antifungal antibiotic and also another antibiotic nystatin (Nystan, Mycostatin—Squibb) is available and useful for their action against this fungus by local application. They are therefore used in intestinal moniliasis. The fungus may pass through the bowel and produce an eruption on the buttocks, treatment for which requires the application of either of these antibiotics in ointment or cream form. The local application of a 1 per cent gentian violet solution may also be successful.

6. *Angular stomatitis.* This condition, also known as perlèche, occurs as fissures and cracks at the angles of the mouth, and is due to deficiency of vitamin B_2 (riboflavin).

7. *Herpangina.* This disease is due to the Coxsackie A virus which produces small vesicles and ulcers on the posterior palate and fauces. It is associated with a pyrexial illness with constitutional changes. There is no specific therapy available; the condition usually improves in about 10 days.

There are other uncommon causes of stomatitis, such as that found in agranulocytosis and in heavy metal poisoning by lead, mercury and bismuth. Cases of pink disease (acrodynia) may also have stomatitis, and in cases of whooping cough a small ulcer of the fraenum below the tongue is occasionally found.

THE TONGUE

The condition of tongue-tie is far less common than has been believed. It is due to a short fraenum which is attached close to the tip of the tongue. In severe cases it may interfere with sucking, but only very, very rarely should it be divided. Geographical tongue occurs, with whitish patches on the tongue giving a map-like appearance. This condition is of no consequence and no treatment is required. A large tongue (macroglossia) is found in cretinism and also due to lymphan-giomatous enlargement.

THE TEETH

There is no doubt that the eruption of teeth in a baby (teething) may be accompanied by mild symptoms, but it is important to stress that teething is a physiological process; all other causes for a child's symptoms must be excluded before blaming this condition. The mild symptoms of teething may include dribbling at the mouth with slight fretfulness. Mild bronchitis or loose stools may also occur in some cases.

Dental caries is an unfortunate and prevalent condition. There are many factors involved and the exact aetiology is not known. Regular dental attention and careful daily oral hygiene are essential in the care of the teeth, in addition to an adequate diet. The fluoridation of drinking water is also a useful method of prevention.

THE OESOPHAGUS

Oesophagitis has already been discussed in relation to thrush infections.

Congenital abnormalities of the oesophagus occur rarely. In these cases there is atresia of the oesophagus with obstruction to its continuity. There may also be a communication between the lower segment of the oesophagus and the trachea, giving rise to the condition of oesophageal atresia with tracheo-oesophageal fistula. This condition presents itself clinically soon after birth with the child bringing up excessive amounts of mucus. In addition, the first feed is brought back and vomited with much frothy material and a cyanotic attack. The condition may be confirmed by the fact that a catheter cannot be passed into the stomach, and also radiology should be used to show a

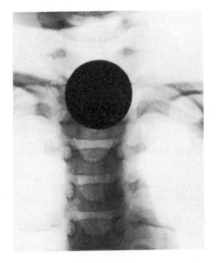

Fig. 6.1 X-ray showing a swallowed coin impacted in the oesophagus.

radio-opaque tube in the oesophagus and with a contrast medium but *not* barium. It is important to recognise the condition as soon as possible after birth so that surgery may be performed in order to save the infant's life. Hydramnios during pregnancy is frequently associated with this condition.

Congenital stenosis of the oesophagus may also occur, giving rise to difficulty in swallowing.

THE STOMACH AND INTESTINES

Colic

This condition may occur in the early months of life and is associated with attacks of violent screaming and abdominal pain. It is probably due to irregular violent intestinal peristaltic movements possibly caused by overfeeding or the excessive use of sugar in the feed. Underfeeding with air-swallowing might also produce colic in infancy. The treatment involves rectifying the cause and using some carminative mixture with a sedative or an antispasmodic such as dicyclomine (Merbentyl).

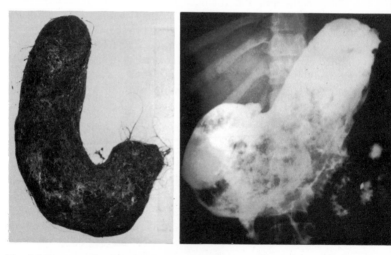

Fig. 6.2 Photograph of a trichobezoar (hairball) successfully removed at operation from the stomach of a 9-year-old girl.
Fig. 6.3 X-ray of the patient with the trichobezoar taken five minutes after the ingestion of barium. The hairball is outlined by the barium in the stomach. (*By courtesy from Friedlander & Kushlick: 'Archives of Disease in Childhood'.*)

Constipation

It should be remembered that a breast-fed infant may have a stool only every second day or less frequently, but these are of normal consistency and are not constipated. Constipation is a symptom, may be due to various causes and is relative to the consistency of the stool rather than the infrequency. The aetiology may be found in the diet, in a lesion of the intestinal tract or in the faulty training of the infant. Underfeeding is probably the commonest cause; there may also be too little sugar in the feed or the child's fluid intake may be too low. The lesions in the lower alimentary tract include such conditions as Hirschsprung's disease or a long kinked pelvic colon. Anal stenosis and anal fissure may cause constipation, while faulty training has also been blamed. In cases of cretinism, mental defect and congenital pyloric stenosis constipation may also be severe; treatment requires an attack on the cause.

In the older age group of childhood, constipation may again be caused by a faulty diet where there is a lack of bulk or a low fluid

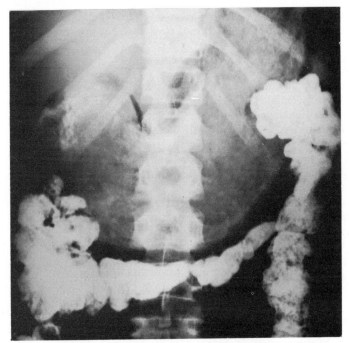

Fig. 6.4 Another X-ray of the same case as Figs 6.2 and 6.3 taken some hours after the ingestion of barium showing the colon well filled with barium still enmeshed in the hairball in the stomach. (*By courtesy from Friedlander & Kushlick: 'Archives of Disease in Childhood'.*)

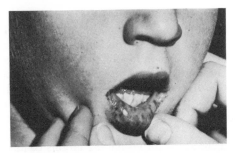

Fig. 6.5 Brown pigmentation of the mucous membrane of the lips and mouth in a child with Peutz-Jeghers syndrome. This is a hereditary dominant condition and may be associated with polyposis of the bowel.

intake, and also lack of exercise. On the other hand, organic conditions of the lower bowel such as those mentioned as occurring in infancy may be the causative factor. But the most important cause in this age group is faulty training and habitual neglect to empty the rectum. In some cases of psychological abnormality constipation may develop when treatment should be in relation to the cause and an attempt made to influence the child's daily routine into regular habits. Drugs may have to be used at the beginning of treatment but not in excess.

Vomiting

Vomiting frequently occurs in infancy. Regurgitation or possetting must be differentiated from true vomiting. The causes of vomiting in infancy may be dietetic in origin and due to such conditions as over-feeding, underfeeding and air-swallowing (aerophagy). Conditions such as congenital hypertrophic pyloric stenosis and pylorospasm are important causes of vomiting. Congenital abnormalities of the oeso-phagus, duodenum (Figs 6.6 and 6.7) and intestine are other causes. Intracranial haemorrhage may also be associated with this symptom, and vomiting may again be symptomatic of other diseases such as acute infections. Rumination and chalasia are also entities in infancy as causes of vomiting (Figs 6.8 and 6.9).

In the older child vomiting may occur in emotional upsets or be symptomatic of some physical disorder; overeating and cyclical vomiting are other causes in the older child. Infections, particularly cerebral conditions, are often associated with vomiting.

Congenital hypertrophic pyloric stenosis

This disease occurs in infancy and produces obstruction to the passage of food from the stomach to the duodenum at the pylorus. It is due to hypertrophy of the circular muscle fibres of the pylorus and is a congenital abnormality.

Aetiology
In this condition the symptoms almost never start at birth, but occur from the second or third week. It is very uncommon for the symptoms to be delayed into the second month. Males are far more commonly affected than females in a proportion of about six to one. It is remark-able that in males the disease seems to affect most commonly the firstborn of a family.

Clinical features
There are five main clinical features making up this condition.

1. *Vomiting.* The vomiting is projectile in nature and is ejected with great force, sometimes coming from the nose as well as from the mouth,

spurting a distance of two to three feet from the infant. At first the vomiting occurs after almost every feed, but later as the stomach becomes more dilated, there may be only one or two large vomits in the day. The vomitus is always acid and never contains bile.

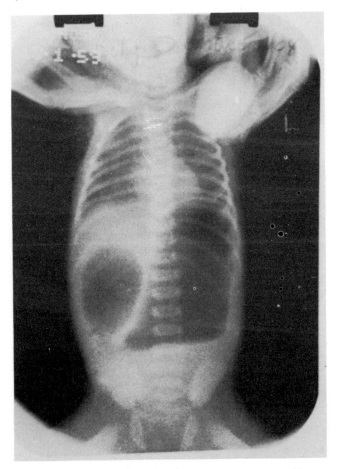

Fig. 6.6 X-ray (erect) of newborn child showing dilatation of the stomach and duodenum with a fluid level and no gas in the lower part of the bowel indicating duodenal obstruction due to congenital atresia.

2. *Constipation.* This is another feature of the condition, but is not always present. It may be pronounced or slight.

3. *Wasting.* Early in the disease the infant's weight may remain stationary, but later declines. The facies of the infant has a worried expression and becomes quite drawn.

4. *Visible peristalsis of the stomach.* This is seen most frequently

after a feed. The waves of peristalsis start at the left costal margin and pass over the epigastrium to fade away on the right side, giving the appearance of a succession of golf balls passing across the upper abdomen.

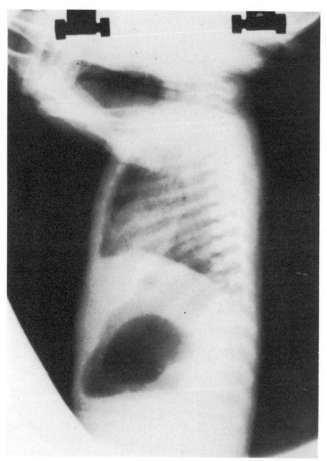

Fig. 6.7 Lateral view of infant in Fig. 6.6.

5. *Presence of a pyloric tumour.* The proper technique must be used in order to feel this mass. The best time to feel the tumour is when the child is being fed, and the examiner should be on the left side of the patient. The examining hand must be warm and must be laid gently on the upper abdomen. The tumour may be felt at a point about midway between the umbilicus and the costal margin at the outer border of the right rectus muscle. This mass is felt to undergo periodic contraction (hardening) and relaxation; patience is required to feel it. It is essential

to feel the tumour in order to substantiate the diagnosis of pyloric stenosis. The differential diagnosis is from pylorospasm and congenital duodenal stenosis; in these conditions, however, the features may be the same, except that the tumour is not present. Furthermore, in duodenal stenosis the symptoms often start soon after birth and the vomitus may be bile-stained.

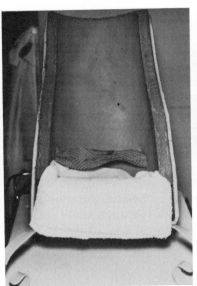 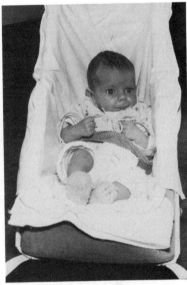

Fig. 6.8 A chair constructed to nurse an infant in the upright posture, suitable for the medical management of cases of hiatus hernia and chalasia with vomiting.
Fig. 6.9 The same chair as in previous figure with a patient in position.

Treatment

The treatment of this condition may be medical or surgical. The preferable method is surgical management. Surgical treatment requires the performance of the Fredet-Ramstedt pyloromyotomy operation. This involves the longitudinal surgical division of the pyloric tumour down to the submucosa. With this method the child may be breast fed again after 48 hours. Medical treatment requires stomach washouts with saline if vomiting is profuse, breast milk or other suitable feeds, intravenous fluids if there be dehydration, and the use of atropine methonitrate (Eumydrin). This drug is used in a 0·6 per cent alcoholic solution or a *freshly* prepared solution of 1 in 1000 in water and is given by mouth 20 minutes before each feed; a 1 in 10,000 solution has also been used in the appropriate larger dose. This drug relaxes the spasm which is a feature of the disease together with the hypertrophied muscle of the pylorus. Many successes follow this method of treatment but prolonged hospitalisation (with all its disadvantages) may be necessary. Another drug, methylscopolamine nitrate (Skopyl), has also been used instead of atropine methonitrate.

Pylorospasm responds very well to this same medical treatment.

Rumination

This condition is also known as merycismus. There is a regurgitation of milk from the stomach into the mouth; this milk is chewed, tasted and then reswallowed. It is found only in artificially fed infants over the age of about 4 months. The child seems to derive much pleasure from the procedure but on each occasion some of the milk spills out of the mouth and eventually there may be much weight loss and under-nutrition. Fortunately, this is an extremely rare condition, but the habit may be very difficult to treat once it is well established. The feeds should be thickened and the child carefully and adequately nursed. (Useful thickening agents are Nestargel (Nestle) and Carobel (Cow and Gate.)

Chalasia of the lower end of the oesophagus may also cause vomiting in the young infant; these cases improve by being nursed in an upright posture. Vomiting may also occur with constipation and a failure to thrive in the rare diseases of renal acidosis and idiopathic hyper-calcaemia which are briefly discussed elsewhere in this book.

Acute diarrhoeal disorders of infancy

Infantile diarrhoea is still, unfortunately, a very common condition and a threat to infant life. In the past this condition was occasionally caused by errors in the diet such as too much sugar or starch or fat intolerance. Infections in situations outside the alimentary system were in the past also associated with diarrhoea. These parenteral infections included otitis media, upper respiratory infections and pyelitis and with their rapid response to treatment are not usually associated with diarrhoea. The main cause of infantile diarrhoea is infection of the bowel and these cases of infective diarrhoea may be caused by a specific organism such as those of the dysenteric group (e.g. *Shigella sonnei* or *flexneri*) or various strains of the Salmonella organism. These cases have diarrhoea often with blood and mucus in the stools, and respond well to the sulpha drugs or antibiotics such as ampicillin. Many of these cases may be due to one of the specific pathogenic serotypes of *Escherichia coli* (e.g. 0111; B 4) and it is these types which may spread to other infants in close contact such as in a hospital ward. Viruses of various types have also been incriminated as a cause of infantile diarrhoea.

Clinical features

These patients all have loose, frequent, green stools and occasionally there is some vomiting. For convenience, these cases may be divided into those with dehydration and those without. The group without dehydration respond well to dietetic treatment, but the group with dehydration are much more seriously ill. In addition to being dehydrated, they may become acidotic and toxic, when urgent therapy becomes necessary. The infant, therefore, with dehydration and acidosis must be clinically recognised. These infants have a sunken fontanelle, dry skin and dry mucosal surfaces of the mouth and tongue. The skin loses its elasticity (tissue turgor) and in the acidotic toxic patient the eyes become sunken and the breathing rapid.

Treatment

Cases with dehydration require urgent treatment to replace their water loss and to correct electrolyte dysbalance. Any infection must also be treated. The infants not seriously ill may be given oral half-strength saline, but those more severely ill require preferably intravenous fluid therapy, or if this is not possible, subcutaneous fluids with the use of hyaluronidase to aid absorption. The initial fluid should be given in the form of half-strength saline, Ringer lactate solution or other appropriate electrolyte solution, followed by 5 per cent dextrose in water. The infant requires 150 ml of fluid per kg bodyweight per 24 hours; this should be made up of approximately 30 to 50 ml per kilo bodyweight of the appropriate electrolyte solution followed by 5 per cent dextrose in water, to make up the total requirements of 150 ml per kg in the 24 hours. In addition, on the first day of treatment, the infant requires an additional amount of about 200 to 300 ml of fluid to make up his fluid loss. A great deal of attention has been focused on the question of low blood potassium levels (hypopotassaemia) being one of the causes of severe illness in cases of acute diarrhoeal disorders in infancy; in this connection solutions such as Darrow's for intravenous therapy are very useful on account of their potassium content, but it must be remembered that intravenous potassium therapy must be undertaken with care as it has certain dangers. Feeding may be started as soon as the vomiting has ceased and half-strength saline may be used at first followed by diluted skimmed milk preparations. This feed should be gradually increased in strength until the child is back to its normal feeding schedule. Antibiotics may be useful in certain cases.

Some infants who are extremely ill may profit from a plasma or small blood transfusion.

Rare conditions associated with diarrhoea and failure to thrive may be due to bowel enzyme deficiencies not allowing proper digestion of carbohydrates such as lactose, sucrose, isomaltose and maltose. In these diseases the enzymes such as lactase, sucrase, isomaltase and maltase may be deficient.

Ulcerative colitis

This is a chronic disease of the large bowel and is rare in children. In this condition there is general wasting and malaise and the main symptom is a continuing diarrhoea with blood in the stools. Confirmation of the diagnosis may be made by sigmoidoscopy and barium enema studies. Some of these cases respond to salicylazosulphapyridine (sulphasalazine, Salazopyrin) but corticosteroid therapy may be necessary. Major surgical procedures involving colectomy may also be necessary in order to control the disease.

Crohn's disease (regional enteritis or ileitis)

This is a chronic granulomatous disease usually limited to the terminal ileum but it may extend upwards into the jejunum or downwards into the colon. It is unusual in the young but may occur in later childhood. It is usually of slow onset and may suggest a low-grade infection. The symptoms may include periodic fever, recurrent abdominal pain, intermittent constipation, anorexia and diarrhoea with pus, mucus and blood in the stool. There is often loss of weight. External anal fistulae may occur (Fig. 6.10) and other unusual symptoms

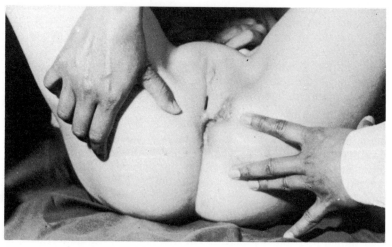

Fig. 6.10 Anal fistula in a child with Crohn's disease.

may include erythema nodosum and clubbing of the fingers. Occasionally a mass may be felt in the abdomen. The erythrocyte sedimentation rate (ESR) may be raised and the serum proteins altered with a reversal of the albumen/globulin ratio. Radiological examination of the bowel with a contrast medium may be helpful and also sigmoidoscopy and colonoscopy. The cause of this condition is unknown and the treatment includes the use of the corticosteroids and also surgical resection of the affected part.

Intestinal parasitic diseases

Threadworm. This worm is known as *Oxyuris vermicularis* and is the commonest intestinal parasite seen in childhood. The worms are small—about 0·5 cm in length—and occur in multitudes, becoming lodged in the caecum and appendix. They lay eggs and pass down to the anus where they cause much perianal irritation. The child scratches himself and in doing so infects his fingers with new ova which are then transferred back to the mouth producing reinfestation. The diagnosis of this condition is best done by using the NIH cellophane swab. This is rubbed on the perianal skin and then transferred to a slide and examined under a microscope for the ova of the worm. Many symptoms have been blamed on this unfortunate worm! Mild ill health and loss of appetite are usual accompanying features of the condition which should be treated although it is difficult to cure. Some cases of vulvovaginitis are due to this worm infestation.

Treatment
Various preparations have been used in the treatment of this condition but probably the most effective drug available is piperazine. This drug, available commercially as Entacyl, Antepar and Pripsen (with senna), is given orally in divided daily dosage for one week. A repeat course is often given after a week to ensure eradication of the threadworm. Another useful drug for the treatment of this condition is a dye preparation known as viprynium embonate (Vanquin) which is used in a single dose of 50 mg per 10 kg bodyweight. This preparation may stain the stools red. Thiabendazole (Mintezol) has also been used but this drug is more effective in eradicating trichiuris infestation (whipworm). It must be remembered, however, that these drugs only supplement, but in no way supersede, the usual hygienic measures which must always be carried out. These are the boiling of the child's underclothing, the cutting short of the nails, the use of cotton gloves at night and very occasionally the application of a dilute mercury ointment around the anus to form a barrier and prevent the worm crossing over to lay its eggs. It is important to remember that there is always the possibility of other members of the same family having the same infestation and, if so, treatment must be prescribed for them.

Roundworm. This worm is known as *Ascaris lumbricoides* and resembles an earthworm in appearance. Only two or three may infest the bowel and although the ova are passed in large quantities they do not give rise to many symptoms. In rare cases, however, there may be so many (hundreds) of these worms present that intestinal obstruction may occur.

The life cycle of this parasite (a nematode) involves the systemic passage of the developing larva. The swallowed ovum hatches in the small bowel; the larva then penetrates the bowel wall and migrates in the circulatory system to the right side of the heart and then, via the pulmonary artery, to the lung where the parasite enters the air sac and passes up the respiratory system to the pharynx where it is swallowed and moves to the small bowel.

Treatment

Piperazine in single dosage is very effective in treating infestations with this worm. Bephenium hydroxynaphthoate (Alcopar) is also effective and especially useful when an additional hookworm infestation is present.

Tapeworm. Tapeworm infestation brought about by the eating of infected pork or infected beef may be caused by two important varieties:

1. *Taenia saginata* (beef tapeworm—'measly' beef)
2. *Taenia solium* (pork tapeworm—'measly' pork)

These worms grow in the bowel to the great length of over 3 metres (10 feet), and the person who has the infestation passes strips of the flat segments of the worm in the stools.

Treatment

The important part of the treatment is to eradicate the head of the worm. The drugs that may be successful in eradicating the tapeworm infestation include niclosamide (Yomesan) and dichlorophen (Antiphen), both of which disintegrate the worm and therefore the head cannot be identified to confirm the cure. The success of treatment is gauged by the absence of recurrence of symptoms in the three months after treatment. In the past the toxic drug *Filix mas* (malefern) was used but this required difficult and inconvenient methods of administration. Mepacrine has also been used in the treatment of tapeworm infestation.

Visceral larval migrans

With certain nematode infections the life cycle in man may allow for the systemic migration of the larvae with serious pathological effects. This is an uncommon condition which may affect children who are infected with the dog roundworm (*Toxocara canis*) or less commonly other nematodes (e.g. the cat roundworm—*Toxocara cati*, or *Capillaria hepatica*). A triad of symptoms is usually found in these patients; these include hepatomegaly (enlarged liver), eosinophilia (increased blood eosinophils) and a history of dirt eating (pica). The patient is usually severely ill and the diagnosis may be confirmed by liver biopsy; serological tests and also a skin test are available for the diagnosis of

Toxocara infestation. The liver appears to be a common site for the deposition of the migrating larvae but other areas such as the eye might also be involved. Treatment with diethylcarbomazine (Banocide) or thiabendazole (Mintezol) may be effective.

Giardiasis

This is an infestation of the small bowel with the protozoon *Giardia lamblia*. This organism may be found in the stool as a flagellate or in their cystic form. If the infestation is severe it may cause diarrhoea, which may occur as steatorrhoea with bulky pale stools containing mucus. It responds very well to therapy with oral mepacrine. This drug should be given for a five-day period in a dosage appropriate to the age of the child. Metronidazole (Flagyl) may also be used.

Amoebiasis

This is a protozoan infection usually of the large bowel that produces a dysentery. The infecting agent is the protozoon *Entamoeba histolytica*. The infection may also spread to the liver, producing an amoebic abscess of that organ. It is common in certain tropical and subtropical areas of the world. The dysentery is associated with frequent stools containing blood and mucus. It is a difficult condition to treat although very effective drugs are available. Emetine is still used in the severely ill and is effective and combined with another amoebacide preparation such as metronidazole (Flagyl). Diloxanide furoate, diodohydroxy-quinoline (Diodoquin) and paromomycin (Humatin) are also used.

Cyclical vomiting (periodic syndrome)

This is a condition associated with vomiting in the young child; it may be accompanied by prostration and severe illness. It occurs in regular attacks and usually disappears by puberty. The child is usually of a highly strung nervous nature and is used to eating a high fat diet. There may be intense vomiting and abdominal pain; the pain, however, follows the vomiting and the abdomen is not distended. There are ketone bodies in the urine. The treatment involves giving large quantities of fluids with glucose in addition to sedating the child. The subsequent management of these cases requires a low fat, high carbohydrate diet and the management of the psychoemotional stress situation.

Steatorrhoea and malabsorption

This condition occurs as a symptom of many different diseases, and is often associated with a failure to thrive. The patient passes large, bulky, fatty, pale, malodorous stools and the term malabsorption is usually used. Amongst the causes of the condition may be:

1. Coeliac disease
2. Cystic fibrosis (fibrocystic disease of the pancreas, muco-viscidosis)

These are the most important causes of the malabsorption syndrome with steatorrhoea and a failure to thrive and will be discussed in more detail.

Less frequent causes are:

3. Post-diarrhoeal conditions
4. Drug-induced enteropathy (e.g. neomycin)
5. Massive infestation of the small bowel with the protozoal organism *Giardia lamblia*
6. Conditions producing interference to the processes of fat absorption, such as abdominal tuberculosis, which may block the lacteals and so prevent fat absorption
7. Congenital duodenal abnormality with partial obstruction
8. Disaccharide enzyme deficiencies (e.g. lactase, sucrase-isomaltase)
9. Very rare possibilities include an abnormality of the lymphatic vessels of the bowel (lymphangiectasia) with a protein-losing enteropathy; a skin condition associated with similar bowel symptoms (acrodermatitis enteropathica) and also the condition of a-β-lipoproteinaemia in which abnormally shaped red blood cells with sharp projections (acanthocytes) are found

Coeliac disease

The original description of this condition was made by Samuel Gee and it is a definite disease entity. The clinical features of the condition are made up of:

1. Anorexia. The child develops a marked anorexia for most foods and there is extreme difficulty in getting the patient to take any diet.
2. Age of onset. This condition seldom occurs before the sixth month and frequently starts between the sixth and ninth months.
3. Failure to thrive. This is a marked feature of the condition, and there is much loss of weight with wasting. This wasting character-istically first affects the buttocks and then the limbs and trunk with the face being involved last of all.
4. Abdominal distension. This is an early sign of the disease and remains as a feature throughout the illness. It is, however, a feature of other types of malabsorption conditions.
5. Altered behaviour. These children, from having an extremely happy disposition, become very morose and disinterested. They are very irritable and have temper attacks. This interesting behaviour change

occurs in all these cases and appears to be the first thing which improves in these patients. The intelligence is not affected.

6. The stools. The stools are characteristically fatty, bulky, pale and malodorous. They may not be frequent but are as a rule very large. The fat content of these stools is increased and this can be determined by the laboratory. Undigested starch granules may also be present.

7. Miscellaneous symptoms. The deficiency states may occur in this disease; these may affect the various vitamins. The serum proteins may also be low, giving rise to oedema.

Radiological examination of the gastrointestinal tract with a barium meal shows clumping of the barium in the small intestine; this feature, however, is characteristic of other malabsorption conditions. The glucose tolerance curve in these cases is usually of the 'flat' type, with the blood sugar never rising more than 40 mg per cent during the test. A necessary investigation of these cases of malabsorption is the D-xylose absorption test. This substance is normally absorbed in the upper small bowel and in certain malabsorption problems the lack of proper absorption can be estimated with this test. Five g of D-xylose is given by mouth and the excretion measured in the urine over a five-hour period; normal absorption is indicated by values of 25 per cent or more of the ingested dose being excreted in the urine in the five-hour period whereas values below 15 per cent indicate malabsorption with an equivocal range between these two levels. The pancreatic enzymes are normal in this condition, in contrast to cystic fibrosis, although some authorities have recorded low levels of amylase in the pancreatic secretions in coeliac disease. The blood picture may show a hypochromic anaemia. An essential investigation in cases of coeliac disease is the examination of the mucosa of the small bowel and specimens for examination are obtained by the technique of peroral aspiration of the duodenojejunal mucosa using the Crosby-Kugler capsule or its modification. This technique may have complications such as perforation of the bowel or haemorrhage and careful observation of the patient after this test has been performed is necessary. The mucosal biopsy when examined microscopically shows a flattening of the villi in coeliac disease. A similar finding has also been seen in conditions such as giardial infestation, iron-deficiency anaemia or postdiarrhoeal disorders.

In relation to the cause of coeliac disease a link has been found between the ingestion of flours containing gluten as a causative factor and these cases may also be known as gluten-induced enteropathy which is a synonymous term to coeliac disease. Wheat and rye flour contain gluten, but corn flour does not, and success has followed the exclusion of gluten from the diet in these cases. In order to exclude such gluten these children may have corn flour in place of the usual wheat. Gluten-free foods are available for the proper management of these children. The basic treatment of this condition is mainly dietetic, and requires the use of a simple diet initially containing such foods as skimmed cow's milk with added glucose and protein and bananas. This diet may be gradually increased but must remain gluten-free; success is obtained after much patience and time has been expended. In addition, the vitamins must be given in adequate dosage and careful treatment and reassessment is necessary to assess normal growth in these patients. In the untreated or partially treated condition growth may be retarded. Cases of coeliac disease have a tendency to become rapidly dehydrated and these acute phases must be urgently treated with the use of intravenous infusions including plasma. In the well controlled patient the atrophy of the villi regenerates and ultimately becomes normal.

Cystic fibrosis (fibrocystic disease of the pancreas, mucoviscidosis)

This is not a true cystic disease; it affects the exocrine portion of the pancreas only but not the endocrine part (the islets of Langerhans); therefore diabetes mellitus is not a feature of the disease although it may be a complication in a few cases (5 per cent). The exocrine portion secretes the pancreatic enzymes—amylase (starch-splitting), trypsin (protein-splitting) and lipase (fat-splitting). In this disease these digestive enzymes are partially or completely absent and the symptomatology is based on this lack, although there is an additional important feature in the condition in that all the mucus-secreting glands such as those of the bronchi produce a thick, viscid secretion, giving the term mucoviscidosis as another name to describe this disease. This fact also explains other important clinical features of this condition.

Clinical features

In the newborn period this disease may occasionally present itself as an intestinal obstruction associated with thick, viscid plugs of meconium (meconium ileus). The infant may show the usual signs of intestinal obstruction such as vomiting and abdominal distension; radiological examination is necessary to confirm the diagnosis. The X-ray examination requires erect views of the abdomen to be studied, which show the distended loops of bowel with the fluid levels usually seen in intestinal obstruction. On rare occasions, the bowel may perforate and the condition will then be complicated by the development of meconium peritonitis, which would show peritoneal calcification on radiological examination of the abdomen. These neonatal conditions require urgent surgical intervention or may be relieved by using bowel washouts with Gastrografin. If the newborn phase is passed without symptoms, as frequently happens, the disease may present itself soon after and develop into the full-blown entity.

The clinical features are best described as relative to three main groups of symptoms:

1. *Alimentary symptoms.* These symptoms include the typical fatty steatorrhoeal stools, and are associated with the absence of the pancreatic enzymes. The appetite in this condition is excellent such that these infants may be ravenous—this is in marked contrast to the extreme anorexia of coeliac disease. The abdomen becomes distended as is found in coeliac disease. Rectal prolapse may occur.
2. *Respiratory symptoms.* These cases often develop respiratory symptoms giving rise to recurrent attacks of bronchitis, bronchopneumonia and bronchiectasis; lung abscesses may also occur. The responsible organism most frequently found is the *Staphylococcus aureus*, although other organisms are also often present. In the initial stages the respiratory symptoms may present as a spasmodic cough simulating whooping cough (pertussis). These symptoms are probably related to the thick secretions from the mucus-secreting glands with secondary bacterial infection with *Staphylococcus aureus* and other organisms. Nasal polyps may be found in these children.
3. *Nutritional symptoms.* These patients show a marked failure to thrive, which is surprising in view of their large appetites. They develop wasting in the same way as in coeliac disease, this being most marked in the buttocks. The abdomen, as already mentioned, becomes distended and evidence of other nutritional deficiency states relative to the vitamins may develop.

It is known that there is a familial basis for this disease in that the siblings of a patient may also develop the same condition. The genetic transmission is on an autosomal recessive basis with a 25 per cent risk to the siblings of a patient having the same condition.

The pancreatic enzymes are absent. In the past it was necessary to confirm the diagnosis by demonstrating this absence by the technique of duodenal intubation thereby obtaining duodenal secretions which were tested for the presence or absence of trypsin, using the gelatine-digestion test. The duodenal juice which is normally clear, mucoid, alkaline, not too viscid and light yellowish in colour is found in this disease to be extremely viscid and sparse with absent or low tryptic activity. If the trypsin was absent it was concluded that the other pancreatic enzymes were also not present. The stools may be tested for the presence or absence of trypsin; its absence may be a good indication of the disease in infants under a year of age. A *fresh* specimen of stool must always be tested, but it must be stressed that the stool test for trypsin may be misleading as gelatine may be digested by proteolytic organisms in the stool, even in the absence of trypsin. It has been demonstrated that the sweat of these patients has a higher than normal content of sodium and chloride. This fact of the high salt content of sweat in patients with cystic fibrosis has provided an excellent means of confirming the diagnosis in suspected cases (abnormal results require that the level of sodium be above 60 mmol per litre). The collection of sweat by the iontophoretic method of ionising pilocarpine on the skin and the estimation of the sodium content in the sweat serves as an excellent method of confirming the diagnosis of this disease. A clinical result of this high salt content of sweat renders these patients liable to develop the effects of heatstroke in hot weather when they lose excessive amounts of salt in their sweat. Saliva also has this raised electrolyte level and methods of estimating the sodium level are available; raised levels of sodium are also found in the nails. A glucose tolerance curve in these patients may be normal or 'flat'. The fat content of the stool, as in coeliac disease, is increased and this abnormality of fat absorption may be proved by estimating the fat content of stools collected for a reasonably long period of time (72 hours or longer). A fat balance test may also be done by giving the child a known amount of fat over a period of time and measuring the quantity excreted in the stools; a normal child taking 25 g of fat per day should not excrete more than 2 g under normal circumstances. The increased excretion of fat is the same in both coeliac disease and cystic fibrosis. Other methods of testing fat absorption have also been done such as the absorption of a fat-soluble substance such as vitamin A given orally, but these tests are not necessary. In cases of cystic fibrosis there is an increased excretion of nitrogen in the stool due to the lack of trypsin. Males with cystic fibrosis will become aspermic and sterile. In the newborn meconium may have a raised albumin content and this fact is the basis of a screening test for this disease in the newborn period. This test is performed on meconium passed by the infant. The BM (Boehringer-Mannheim) meconium test makes use of a paper strip dipped into a solution of meconium and assessing a possible colour change. In positive cases an intense blue colour develops in the test strip above the meconium. These cases would require further assessment with the sweat test.

Treatment

The basis of the treatment of cystic fibrosis is aimed at improving and maintaining nutrition and preventing and treating the pulmonary condition. The treatment is long term and it is extremely important that an adequate follow-up of patients be arranged. The pulmonary infection, which is the main cause of death in these cases, must be prevented if possible or kept under control by maintenance antibiotic therapy using a suitable broad-spectrum antibiotic on a continuous basis or actively treating any pulmonary infection as it arises. It is useful to obtain sputum at intervals for bacteriological examination and sensitivity tests to various antibiotics in order that more adequate control of bacterial infection be obtained. Postural drainage is essential in clearing mucus secretions and physiotherapy may be extremely helpful in this respect. The use of acetylcysteine (Airbron, Mucomyst) administered as an aerosol may be useful in reducing the viscosity of the mucus and helping remove the thick secretions from the bronchi. Aerosol therapy may usefully also have appropriate antibiotics added. If cardiac failure develops, the usual treatment for this is necessary. The dietetic control is important and in addition to this, pancreatic enzymes may be supplied in the form of 'pancreatin' as enteric-coated capsules, powder or granules (Cotazym, Pancrex V); this enteric coating is important as the pancreatic enzymes are inactivated by the gastric juices. The administration of these digestive enzymes controls the stools and the bowel situation is generally improved. Vitamins must be supplied in sufficient quantity and use may also be made of predigested foods such as protein hydrolysates. The medium chain triglycerides (Trufood MCT oil, Mead Johnson MCT oil) may be useful and is also available as a powder (Trufood MCT 1, Mead Johnson Portagen). They do not require pancreatic lipase or bile for their absorption in contrast to the usual long-chain fats normally present in the diet. They may be useful in different malabsorption syndromes such as cystic fibrosis, severe coeliac disease, liver disease, the rare a-β-lipoproteinaemia and other conditions.

The prognosis in this chronic disease is serious and requires careful and adequate control. The most important element in the control is the prevention of the respiratory involvement or if this should occur the proper and careful management of this aspect of the disease. There is a wide range of severity of this disease.

THE LIVER

Jaundice in the neonatal period has already been discussed in a previous section.

Infective hepatitis

This disease is the commonest cause of jaundice in the older child and is due to a virus infection producing hepatitis (viral hepatitis type A). This virus is excreted in the stools and urine of patients and infection may be transmitted by contamination, and also possibly by flies. The incubation period is about 30 days. A similar condition known as homologous serum jaundice with hepatitis (viral hepatitis type B) is transmitted by transfusion or injections where the virus is present in these agents, but may also be transmitted directly by close contact and orally. In these cases the incubation period is longer, being about 100 days. An antigen (Australia antigen) has been identified in the serum of patients with this disease and this is of importance in the identification of the causative virus. It is believed to be closely associated or identical with the virus of this disease.

Clinical features

The illness may start with nausea and vomiting, and also on occasion with severe abdominal pain. There is a pyrexia associated with the illness, and jaundice then appears. This is first noticed in the conjunctivae and later in the skin; it gradually deepens and later fades until it finally disappears. The urine at first is very dark with bile pigment; the stools may be pale. Investigation of the blood shows a rise in the serum bilirubin level and abnormality of the liver function tests. The liver is enlarged and becomes tender. The disease usually improves in a few weeks, but the recovery phase with convalescence may be very prolonged. The outlook in this disease is good, although in very rare cases the hepatitis may go on to fibrosis, with eventual cirrhosis of the liver developing.

Treatment

There is no specific treatment for the disease; the most important feature in its management is absolute bed rest for a long period until the patient is clinically well and the urine becomes completely normal with regard to the excretion of urobilin and urobilinogen; the blood should also have a normal serum bilirubin content. Dietary control is practised; this may be fat-free with a high carbohydrate and protein content although dietary fat is thought not to be harmful in hepatitis. Additional substances of the vitamin B complex group should also be given. Other substances such as arginine, methionine, choline and inositol have been given to these patients but it must be stressed that they are not specific therapy for this disease. In very severe cases, which are complicated by hepatic failure and hepatic coma, it is necessary to restrict protein and to sterilise the bowel with an antibiotic such as neomycin. Steroid administration with ACTH or a cortisone derivative such as prednisone has also been used in the treatment.

Contacts of a case may be protected by passive immunisation with human immunoglobulin.

Cirrhosis of the liver

This is extremely rare in childhood, and the various types as in adults may occur. There may be the biliary type which may follow atresia of the bile ducts or the rare portal cirrhosis. Congenital syphilis may also produce cirrhosis of the liver of the pericellular type.

Reye's syndrome

This condition was described by Reye in 1963 and usually affects infants or small children. The symptoms are rapid in their onset and are associated with an acute and often fatal encephalopathy with abnormal liver function and the development of a severe hypoglycaemia. The cause has not been determined but a viral infection is a possibility. The liver is known to become extremely fatty and show the histological picture of fatty infiltration.

7. Diseases of the Respiratory System

In the early embryo the mouth and nose form a single cavity and this becomes divided by certain processes which unite and fuse to form the palate which separates the nasal and oral cavities. A septum grows down medially to fuse with the palate and form the nasal septum. There are four nasal accessory sinuses, two being present at birth—the maxillary antra and the ethmoids—the sphenoidal sinus is present from the age of about 3 years and the frontal sinuses appear at about 5 years of age, although there is considerable variation. The nasal cavity of the sinuses is lined by ciliated epithelium and mucus-secreting glands open on the surface producing mucus which is propelled towards the nasopharynx. The sense of smell is achieved by air reaching the olfactory nerves in the upper third of the nasal cavity. The nose acts as a filtering agent and air is also warmed as it passes the nasal mucosa. Acute infection of the nasal cavity is most often caused by the common cold (coryza) and this acute rhinitis is important in relation to its association with secondary infection and possible spread to neighbouring parts. Chronic rhinitis may be associated with a bloodstained discharge, the commonest cause of which, if unilateral, is a foreign body which the child has placed in his nose. Another rare cause, in an unimmunised community, of a bloodstained nasal discharge is nasal diphtheria which is usually associated with excoriation below the nostril; in such suspected cases a nasal swab must always be taken. The symptom of 'snuffles' may occur in such conditions as acute rhinitis, Down's syndrome (mongolism), congenital syphilis and congenital enlargement of the adenoids. Acute infections of the nasal accessory sinuses may occur as a spread from the nasopharynx. These infections may be accompanied by pain and some temperature. Chronic infections of the sinuses are more common in childhood and are associated with a blockage of their ostia draining into the nasal cavity. Sinusitis often accompanies the condition of bronchiectasis. Nasal drops such as ephedrine in normal saline may be useful in the treatment of these conditions.

Allergic rhinitis

This condition, also known as hayfever, is very common in allergic subjects. It is due to an inhaled agent such as pollen or housedust and gives rise to frequent periodic attacks of sneezing accompanied by a profuse watery discharge from the nose and also by lachrymation. The antihistamine drugs are useful agents in the treatment of this condition; in addition an attempt should be made to find the cause and remove it if possible. Skin tests might be helpful in some cases in determining the causative agent. Another useful method of treatment is the insufflation into each nostril of *sodium chromoglycate* (Rynacron); this has an effect in inhibiting the release of histamine from the nasal cells. Nasal polypi may develop in patients who have longstanding hayfever and surgery may be required. Some children may gradually improve but many do develop some other allergic disorder such as asthma.

Epistaxis

Epistaxis or nose bleeding is common in childhood and may have a variety of causes, the commonest being local trauma. Certain blood diseases such as purpura, leukaemia and aplastic anaemia may produce epistaxis. Some infections such as typhoid fever may be associated with epistaxis and also rheumatism. It may also occur in mitral heart disease. The treatment should be to stop the bleeding by the usual simple methods but if these fail the anterior or posterior nares may have to be plugged.

THE EARS

Otitis media

The middle ear may be affected with an acute otitis media. It should be remembered that in young infants the Eustachian tube is relatively short and lies horizontally. This fact may allow infection to spread easily from the nasopharynx to the middle ear, with the production of an acute otitis media. This condition in young infants may produce a severe illness with a high temperature. The child may indicate the pain in his ear by constantly pulling at it and there is often irritability, crying and vomiting. On examination, the eardrum is found to be red and inflamed, and may be bulging with pus.

Treatment

The treatment of the condition requires the use of penicillin or other appropriate antibiotic. It is only in rare cases that surgical incision of the drum need be done (myringotomy). The middle ear may become filled with tenacious fluid (glue ear); these patients respond to the insertion of a small Teflon grommet in the eardrum for ventilation. This grommet usually extrudes itself in six to nine months.

Mastoiditis

The mastoids may be infected as a spread from the middle ear, in which case there is pain and swelling of the mastoid region. It responds well to antibiotic therapy and only in neglected cases is surgical inter-vention required. In chronic infections of the ear the drum is usually perforated, giving rise to a chronic discharge. On rare occasions it may be due to tuberculosis and frequently surgical treatment is required.

THE TONSILS AND ADENOIDS

Acute tonsillitis

This is a common infection in childhood and is usually due to a haemolytic streptococcus. The child has a sore throat and may vomit and feel ill. The throat must be examined in order to make the diagnosis. The tonsils may be flecked with small yellow areas of pus—follicular tonsillitis; this condition must be differentiated from diphtheria.

Treatment

Throat swabs should be taken and examined and the condition should be treated with antibiotics or chemotherapy.

The complications of this infection are:

1. Those occurring by direct spread
2. Those occurring by distant spread

Direct spread. A peritonsillar abscess (quinsy) or a retropharyngeal abscess may occur by direct spread of the infection. Cervical adenitis, otitis media, tracheitis or bronchitis may also follow the tonsillitis.

Distant spread. The haemolytic streptococcal infection of the tonsils may be followed by sensitisation of the patient and the production of acute rheumatic fever or acute nephritis after a period of about 10 to 14 days.

Tonsillectomy

Definite indications should be present before the tonsils and adenoids are removed. The commonest indication for this operation is recurrent attacks of sore throat in a child of school-going age. Enlarged tonsils which produce obstruction to breathing is also an indication for the operation. Where quinsy has occurred the tonsils should also be subsequently removed when the acute infection has subsided. In cases of tuberculous cervical adenitis it may also be advisable to perform a tonsillectomy. The diphtheria carrier state might also lead to this operation in order to remove the infecting organisms, where other methods have failed, although penicillin and erythromycin are often successful. In cases of juvenile rheumatism and nephritis, tonsillectomy should only be performed if the usual indications are present. In the presence of an epidemic of poliomyelitis, tonsillectomy should never be performed because of the danger of bulbar poliomyelitis developing in such a patient. Widespread poliomyelitis immunisation, however, has made this disease a rarity.

THE LARYNX

The larynx may be involved by various affections in children with the production of difficult and noisy breathing, i.e. stridor or croup. Stridors may be produced by the following conditions:

1. Diphtheria (laryngeal).
2. Acute laryngitis which may follow a common cold or measles.
3. Laryngismus stridulus. This condition is due to spasm of the laryngeal muscles and occurs in cases of rickets, usually accompanied by tetany and sometimes convulsions. It is due to a low ionic calcium content in the blood.
4. Laryngitis stridulosa. This condition occurs in childhood, when the patient usually awakens suddenly at night with acute laryngeal spasm. It is associated with an infection and responds well to treatment with steam and antibiotics, in addition to sedation to overcome apprehension in the child.
5. Congenital laryngeal stridor. This condition occurs from birth and is due to a congenital narrowing of the larynx. As the child grows the larynx also grows and the condition improves. It is of importance only in so far that superadded infection may produce a dangerous situation.
6. An inhaled foreign body. Urgent treatment is necessary to remove this. The condition as it affects the bronchus and lung will be discussed later.
7. Papilloma. This is an uncommon condition of the larynx, but if present, may produce noisy stridulous breathing.
8. Acute laryngotracheobronchitis. This is an acute inflammatory condition of high virulence with a high mortality rate possibly caused by a virus infection. It is associated with obstruction to breathing by thick plugs of mucus and also spasm. The symptoms include restlessness, anxiety, increasing pulse rate, rib recession, stridor and exhaustion. Treatment is urgently necessary and oxygen should be supplied with moisture; a mucus-loosening agent such as acetylcysteine (Airbron) may be useful. Antibiotics are also necessary and the corticosteroids may be helpful. Tracheostomy should not be considered in the majority of these cases but may be life-saving in some where its use is particularly related to efficient suction of the obstructing mucus from the respiratory tract.
9. Epiglottitis. In this condition the epiglottis is mainly involved usually by infection with type B *Haemophilus influenzae*. The child,

most often between 2 and 6 years of age, becomes rapidly prostrated and extremely ill and has a swollen red epiglottis which has the appearance of a cherry obstructing the pharynx. Ampicillin is the antibiotic of choice and tracheostomy may be life-saving in certain cases.

Less common conditions producing stridor are such rarities as a retrosternal goitre and possibly a double aortic arch. Steam is a very useful agent in most cases of laryngeal stridor.

THE BRONCHI

Acute bronchitis

This occurs most commonly at the extremes of life, i.e. in the young infant and in the elderly patient. It usually follows an upper respiratory

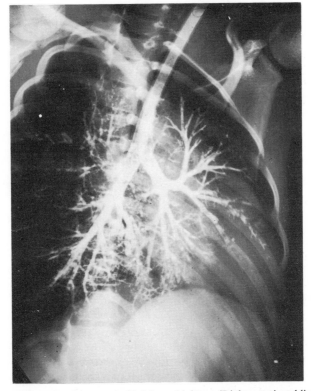

Fig. 7.1 A bronchogram showing a normal left bronchial tree. (Right anterior oblique view.)

infection and may be associated with measles and whooping cough. In the young infant there is obstruction to the breathing with spasm and infection; there is also breathlessness, pyrexia and cyanosis. The infection may spread down into the smaller bronchioles (bronchiolitis);

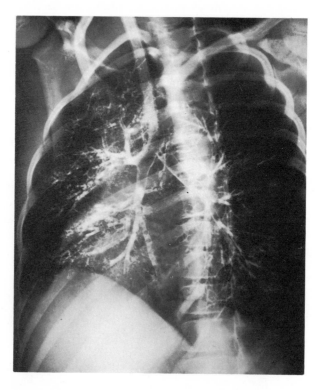

Fig. 7.2 A bronchogram showing some degree of bronchiectasis of the right side. (Left anterior oblique view.)

there is then difficulty in differentiating this condition from broncho-pneumonia. Oxygen is often necessary in the treatment, together with antibiotics.

Chronic bronchitis

These patients have a persistent cough which is usually worse at night and in the early morning. It is always associated with upper respiratory infection and with sinusitis. Tuberculosis, bronchiectasis and inhaled foreign bodies must be differentiated from chronic bronchitis.

Bronchiectasis

This condition is due to a dilatation of the bronchi and is associated with a stagnation of secretions leading to infection. It is usually due to some degree of atelectasis (collapse) of a part of the lung. Fibrosis may also play some part in the production of bronchiectasis. Patchy areas of atelectasis may follow an attack of whooping cough, and this in turn may be followed by bronchiectasis. The clinical picture is made up of a chronic cough, with the production of offensive sputum, mainly in the morning, and the liability to frequent attacks of pneumonia. The dangers are secondary infection, with the production of an abscess in the lung or a spread to the brain producing a cerebral abscess. Radiological examination with the use of contrast medium (bronchogram) is essential in confirming the diagnosis (Fig. 7.2).

Treatment

The treatment may be medical or surgical. Medical treatment involves the use of postural drainage with slapping of the chest to help bring up the secretions, and also breathing exercises. The sinuses are usually infected in this condition and must always be treated. If medical treatment does not succeed, surgical removal of the affected part (lobectomy) is the best means of eradicating the disease.

Inhaled foreign body

It is not uncommon for children to inhale a foreign body such as a peanut. The immediate reaction is for the child to have a coughing spell with a possible 'blue' attack. As the foreign body lodges further down the respiratory tract, the child revives and appears fairly normal. However, on examination of such a patient both clinically and radiologically, evidence may be found of the effects of the inhaled foreign body. It may produce collapse of the part of the lung distal to the bronchus in which it is situated, or it may allow air into this part of the lung without allowing it out (ball-valve effect); this gives the appearance of emphysema of an obstructive nature in the affected part (Fig. 7.3). Urgent bronchoscopic removal of the foreign body under general anaesthesia is necessary in these cases, with the cover of antibiotics. If the foreign body is not removed various complications such as abscess formation or bronchiectasis may arise.

THE LUNGS

Atelectasis

This implies collapse of a part of a lung and may be caused by postoperative blocking of a bronchus with a plug of mucus, inhaled

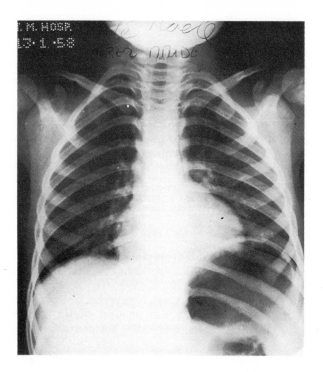

Fig. 7.3 X-ray of chest showing obstructive emphysema of right lung due to an inhaled foreign body.

foreign body or postoperative inhalation of blood following nasal or oral operations. Pressure on a bronchus such as by enlarged tuberculous mediastinal glands may also produce this clinical picture. Fluid or air in the pleura can also collapse a lung by pressure effects (pneumothorax or pleural effusion). The treatment should involve an attack on the cause and an attempt must be made to re-expand the collapsed lung.

Lung abscess

This is uncommon in childhood although it may follow inhalation of a foreign body, pneumonia or atelectasis.

Pneumonia

Acute pneumonic conditions in children may be classified according to their cause, their response to certain drugs or to the area of lung ffected. The last-mentioned is the best method using the classification of lobar pneumonia and bronchopneumonia.

Lobar pneumonia

This condition necessitates hospital treatment much less frequently than in the past on account of the early use of antibiotics. It may occur at any age, but is not common under 1 year. The pathological picture is one of inflammatory exudate filling the alveoli of a lobe of the lung. With improvement this condition clears up entirely leaving a normal lung without fibrosis. This is well demonstrated by X-ray examination (Fig. 7.4). The clinical picture is one of acute illness with fever, vomiting

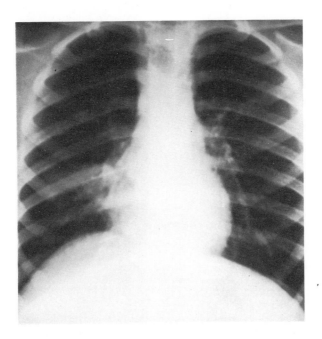

Fig. 7.4 X-ray of chest showing right middle lobe pneumonia.

and occasionally even convulsions. The respiratory rate increases so that the ratio of pulse to the respiratory rate, which is normally four to one, changes to a ratio of two to one. The condition is usually due to a pneumococcus and the pleura may also be involved giving rise to pain. The complications are empyema, lung abscess or acute pneumococcal pericarditis—all extremely rare. Other complications, which occur by blood spread, are meningitis and arthritis. The clinical progress of this disease before the advent of modern therapy was accompanied by a dramatic drop of temperature producing the 'crisis' of the condition. This is not seen at the present time as patients respond rapidly to penicillin or other appropriate antibiotic therapy.

Bronchopneumonia

This condition differs from lobar pneumonia in that it affects lobules of the lung and occurs most commonly under the age of 2 years. It is an inflammatory disease of the bronchioles and the connective tissue between them. Small areas of atelectasis occur, which may not clear up

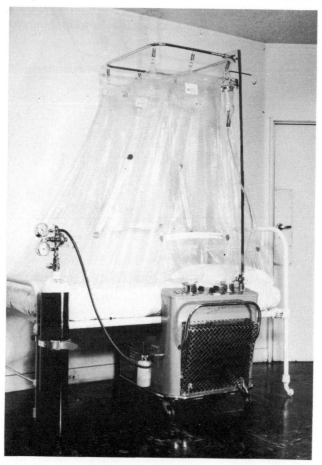

Fig. 7.5 Oxygen tent for bigger children. (*By courtesy of Vickers Ltd.*)

entirely. It is usually due to a pneumococcus but may also be caused by a streptococcus or staphylococcus. It is a disease which complicates other conditions of infancy such as measles, gastroenteritis, whooping cough or any upper respiratory tract infection. The condition is closely related to a bronchiolitis, and the child is extremely ill with fever, breathlessness, active alae nasi, rapid and grunting respirations, restlessness and cyanosis; there is a pause after inspiration instead of after expiration as found normally. Cardiac failure may complicate the clinical picture. The treatment requires careful nursing, oxygen therapy and antibiotics (Figs 7.5 and 7.6). If cardiac failure ensues there is the need to digitalise these patients.

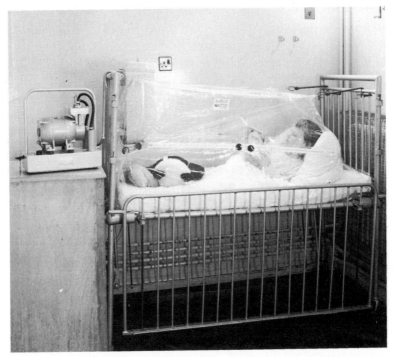

Fig. 7.6 Humidaire tent. (*By courtesy of Vickers Ltd.*)

Staphylococcal pneumonia

This condition may be secondary to any other staphylococcal infection in the body or may be a primary disease; it may affect very young infants (Fig. 7.7). Multiple staphylococcal abscesses appear in the lung, and if one of these is near the pleural surface it may burst into the pleural cavity and produce an empyema. This condition requires careful nursing; it may not respond to penicillin and in this circumstance the synthetic penicillins, such as cloxacillin (Orbenin) or flucloxacillin (Floxapen), or the antibiotics erythromycin, cephaloridine (Ceporin) or sodium fusidate (Fucidin) should be used.

The respiratory infection that occurs in cystic fibrosis is often caused by *Staphylococcus aureus*, as discussed in a previous section.

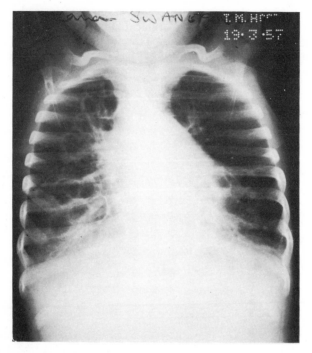

Fig. 7.7 Staphylococcal pneumonia.

Primary atypical pneumonia

This condition producing a pneumonitis is due to the *Mycoplasma pneumoniae* (previously called pleuropneumonia-like organism, PPLO, Eaton agent). This is a small organism without a cell wall which forms small colonies on artificial media. In this disease there is pyrexia with a raised respiratory rate and cough. Radiological examination of the chest shows patchy pneumonic areas and this is helpful in the clinical diagnosis. Ear symptoms may occur in this disease with the development of otitis media and also a bullous haemorrhagic myringitis (affecting the eardrum). A blood count shows a normal or moderately elevated neutrophil white cell count; the blood may contain cold agglutinins but this may also be found in pneumonias due to other viruses, such as the adenoviruses. A useful diagnostic laboratory procedure is the blood complement fixation test. This condition does not respond to penicillin or the sulpha drugs but may respond fairly well to the tetracycline group of antibiotics and also erythromycin. A pneumonitis may also occur in the rickettsial infection known as Q fever due to *Coxiella burnetii*.

Lipoid pneumonia

This disease is found in infants or children who have inhaled an oily substance; it may follow the dangerous practice of forcing oily preparations into children or using oily nasal drops. Paraffin pneumonia or pneumonitis may also occur in children who have accidentally swallowed paraffin when inhalation may occur.

THE PLEURA

Infections of the pleura (pleurisy) may be dry, serous or purulent (empyema). A dry pleurisy complicates pneumonia and gives rise to pain in the chest. A serous pleural effusion may occur in tuberculosis. Empyema may rarely complicate lobar pneumonia and may occur during the attack (synpneumonic) or after the pneumonia (meta-pneumonic). It usually responds very well to appropriate antibiotic therapy.

A bloodstained pleural effusion is rare in childhood, but may be due to trauma or malignant disease.

Pneumothorax (Figs 7.8 and 7.9)

Although this condition may occur in the newborn as a complication of an obstructed bronchus, following the production of an interstitial emphysema, it is rare. Pneumothorax may also occur following the bursting of an emphysematous bulla or a staphylococcal abscess of the lung. It may also be found in whooping cough or following trauma.

Allergic conditions of the respiratory tract

The allergic or hypersensitive reaction of tissues to some foreign material, usually a protein, may manifest itself in various ways. Rhinitis, which has been discussed earlier, may occur. In various nasal conditions infection plays a part but allergy is frequently an additional factor.

Spasmodic asthma is a not uncommon condition in childhood and must be differentiated from asthmatic bronchitis which is due to infection and spasm. Cases of spasmodic asthma are apyrexial, the attack starting and ending suddenly and usually lasting some hours; there is frequently a family history of allergy and the patient may have had other allergic conditions. On the other hand patients with asthmatic bronchitis are pyrexial and have a slow onset of the condition which may last some days.

The aetiology of spasmodic asthma is based on various factors. A constitutional background is often present; these include a family history of allergy and a previous history of some allergic condition in the patient, such as infantile eczema. Extrinsic factors, such as sensi-

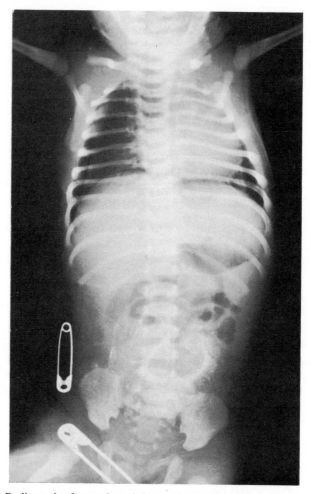

Fig. 7.8 Radiograph of a newborn infant with bilateral pneumothorax producing severe respiratory difficulty with cyanosis.

tivity to various agents, whether inhaled (e.g. pollens) or ingested (e.g. egg, wheat products), are often incriminated as a cause. Intrinsic factors such as psychological stresses are almost always present in the asthmatic child.

Amongst the extrinsic factors there appears to be a relationship between house dust and the house dust mite, of which there are a number of varieties mainly of the genus *Dermatophagoides*. The active allergenic factor in house dust appears to be the mite. This extremely small arthropod thrives on skin particles and is found in houses in

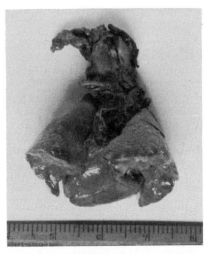

Fig. 7.9 Lungs removed from a newborn infant who died of bilateral pneumothorax. Note the emphysematous bullae over both lungs.

humid, warm conditions mainly in bedding and bedrooms and also other rooms. Vaccines prepared from *D. farinae* are available.

Treatment

In the treatment of this condition an attempt should be made to remove the cause if known, to introduce breathing exercises and to improve the psychological environmental factors. Adrenaline, isoprenaline, salbutamol or aminophylline are used for the acute asthmatic attack and corticosteroid therapy is extremely useful for severe attacks and for status asthmaticus. A substance, disodium cromoglycate (Intal), is available for the better control of this disease and is used on a prophylactic basis. It is available in powder form in capsules for inhalation using a special inhaler (Spinhaler). This substance is available containing a small amount of isoprenaline (Intal Compound) and also without this added (Intal Spincaps). The steroids beclomethasone (Becotide) or betamethasone (Bextasol) as an aerosol may be useful.

Cot Deaths (sudden death syndrome)

This is a fairly common condition of the sudden unexpected and unexplained death of a young infant, previously well, usually between the ages of one month and four months. It occurs most often during the winter months and appears to affect more males than females. Various theories have been put forward as a possible cause. Suffocation by a pillow is a very unlikely cause. Cow's milk sensitisation with anaphylaxis following the aspiration of milk into the air passages may account for a few of these cases but a more likely explanation is an acute respiratory infection and evidence of this may be found at postmortem examination.

8. Tuberculosis

Tuberculosis has been known from early times; in 1882 Robert Koch discovered the tubercle bacillus as being the causative agent.

Tuberculous infection in childhood will be considered under:

1. Intrathoracic tuberculosis
2. Abdominal tuberculosis
3. Miliary tuberculosis and tuberculous meningitis
4. Other forms of tuberculous infection

There are two strains of *Mycobacterium tuberculosis* pathogenic to man, the human type and the bovine type, the former being the more common infecting agent.

Intrathoracic tuberculosis

In childhood intrathoracic tuberculous infection is a different process from that in adults. The disease is caused by the human type of *M. tuberculosis* and infection of the child usually takes place by direct contact with an open case of pulmonary tuberculosis with the inhalation of the infecting organism. The infecting agent lodges in the lung tissue to produce a tubercle; this area of infection is known as the primary focus. The infection spreads back from the primary focus, via the lymphatic vessels, to the draining mediastinal lymph glands. The combination of primary focus (also called a Ghon focus) and the infected lymph glands make up the primary complex of tuberculosis. This primary complex may progress or regress in certain directions:

1. It may heal and eventually calcify
2. The caseous infected glands may press on the neighbouring bronchi and produce atelectasis (collapse) of the lung supplied by that particular bronchus
3. The enlarged gland, in pressing on the bronchus, may act as a ball-valve and allow air into the lung but not out thereby producing the picture of an obstructive emphysema
4. A caseous gland may ulcerate into the bronchus and the infected material may be inhaled into the lung, producing tuberculous bronchopneumonia
5. The gland may ulcerate into a blood vessel and lead to a haematogenous (blood stream) spread of the infection, i.e. miliary tuberculosis.

In addition to these events, the patient may at the same time develop a sensitivity or allergy to the tubercle organism. This may manifest itself in different ways:

(a) By erythema nodosum, a skin condition which is discussed in a later section

(b) By phlyctenular conjunctivitis, an eye condition where small lesions (phlyctenules) appear in the conjunctivae

(c) By a positive Mantoux reaction. The Mantoux test is performed by injecting intradermally 0·1 ml of a 1/1000 solution of old tuberculin or purified protein derivative (PPD) of the tubercle bacillus [which contains 10 tuberculin units (t.u.)]; this is usually injected into the forearm and the test is read after 48 hours have elapsed. A positive reaction is shown by the development of an area of erythema at the injection site. The Heaf multiple puncture test is another satisfactory method as is the Tine tuberculin test (Lederle). The Mantoux reaction itself may also be done in different dilutions, starting with a 1/10,000 solution (containing 1 t.u.), and reducing this gradually if a positive reaction is not obtained, until a 1/100 dilution (containing 100 t.u.) is used, although this strength may give false positive reactions. A positive reaction occurring in a person indicates that that individual has been sensitised to a previous tuberculous infection. As a rule, it takes about six to ten weeks after the primary infection for this allergy to develop. A positive Mantoux reaction in the child under the age of about 3 years probably implies that active tuberculosis is present. In the older child, a positive Mantoux reaction may not be indicative of active disease but of a previous infection which has been overcome. In circumstances with an overwhelming infection such as severe miliary tuberculosis, the Mantoux reaction may become negative.

In the very young child tuberculous infection is a very severe and unfortunate occurrence, and in circumstances where the child develops measles or whooping cough these infections may reactivate a focus of tuberculous infection.

Mediastinal glandular tuberculosis. The enlarged mediastinal glands may produce certain symptoms; of these, the most important is a dry cough. The child may fail to gain weight satisfactorily and have anorexia with a mild pyrexia. However, it must be stressed that the patient with a primary complex may not show any symptoms at all, and the diagnosis can be made only by X-ray examination and a positive Mantoux reaction. The pressure of the enlarged glands on the bronchi may lead to the development of collapse or emphysema, as mentioned previously. If this should occur, the clinical signs of these conditions become manifest.

Tuberculous bronchopneumonia. This condition may develop by a tuberculous gland rupturing into a bronchus. A cough is usually present with much loss of weight, pyrexia and an extremely ill patient. Radiological examination may show fluffy opacities in the lung fields.

Miliary tuberculosis. This condition will be considered in a later section of this chapter.

The diagnosis of tuberculous infection in the chest in childhood is based on a history of previous contact with a case of active open tuberculosis. The clinical findings may be helpful and radiological examination is essential. The Mantoux reaction is extremely important in the diagnosis, and proof of a tuberculous infection may be obtained by finding the organism in the gastric washings of these patients. It is important to realise that young children do not expectorate sputum, but they swallow whatever sputum is produced, and if this contains the tubercle organism it may be found by examining the washings removed from the stomach by tube. Gastric washings should be obtained first thing in the morning, using a saline solution. The prognosis of intrathoracic tuberculosis is far more serious in the young child under the age of 3 years; there is always a risk of the spread of the disease, especially within three months of the primary infection. However, with modern available therapy and excellent child care, the prognosis for eventual recovery is very good.

Treatment

The basic feature of the treatment of these cases is the combination of general care, such as fresh air, adequate periods of rest, an adequate diet, and the use of the antituberculosis drugs. It is acceptable at the present time that the development of a primary tuberculous complex in childhood requires active treatment with a combination of two of the antituberculosis drugs (e.g. INAH and sodium PAS). In the past the primary complex was not actively treated in all children unless sequelae developed from the initial infection. However, in the child under the age of 3 years active treatment is essential; this age may be extended to 5 years and again at other periods of stress such as puberty. It is thought wiser that if a child has a primary tuberculous complex and his health deviates from the normal that child should have active treatment. In this regard the treatment should continue for 6 to 12 months. It is known that the tubercle bacillus has a tendency to develop resistance to the drugs. The dose of streptomycin is 20 to 40 mg per kg bodyweight per day by intramuscular injection; in severe cases such as tuberculous meningitis this may be increased. Isoniazid (INAH) is given orally in an amount of approximately 10 to 20 mg per kg bodyweight per day in divided dosage; this dose may be increased in severe cases. Sodium aminosalicylate (sodium PAS) is also given by mouth and the dosage is about 0·2 g per kg bodyweight per day. Sodium PAS is a useful preparation used in conjunction with the other drug, as it delays the organism developing resistance. In the cases where resistance of the tubercle organism develops to these drugs other antituberculosis preparations such as rifampicin (Rifadin), ethambutol (Myambutol), ethionamide and others are available for use. The usual drugs must be continued for a prolonged period, especially the isoniazid. Streptomycin may produce toxic symptoms such as impaired balance and deafness by its effect on the eighth cranial nerve. INAH has been known to produce rashes and a neuropathy such as peripheral neuritis; the administration of pyridoxine (vitamin B_6) is recommended as a method of preventing this neuropathy.

Abdominal tuberculosis

This type of infection is caused by swallowing the tubercle organism and is usually due to the bovine type of *Mycobacterium tuberculosis* which has its origin in infected cow's milk. With the increased care in the handling of milk and pasteurisation this type of infection is rare. This form of tuberculosis may also be due to the human type bacillus. The infection may affect:

1. The bowel wall (tuberculous enteritis)
2. The mesenteric glands (tabes mesenterica)
3. The peritoneum (tuberculous peritonitis)

Tuberculous enteritis. Ulceration of the lower end of the small intestine may be produced by tuberculous infection. The ulcers spread around the bowel rather than along the length of the bowel as in typhoid fever. The onset may be rather slow and a persistent diarrhoea occurs with blood in the stools. There is wasting, toxaemia, some abdominal pain and pyrexia may be present.

Tabes mesenterica. Tuberculosis usually affects the mesenteric glands in the right iliac fossa and several glands may be involved with the caseous tuberculous process. These glands may eventually heal with fibrosis and calcification. The clinical picture associated with this condition is attacks of pain, with tiredness and loss of weight. There may be diarrhoea with fatty stools (steatorrhoea). The enlarged glands may be felt by palpating the abdomen. Attacks of partial intestinal obstruction may occur.

Tuberculous peritonitis. The peritoneum may be affected in two ways, either with the production of an effusion giving the ascitic type, or with the formation of fibrous tissue with adhesions between the bowel, giving the plastic type of tuberculous peritonitis. In the ascitic variety the abdomen is enlarged, and free fluid can be detected in the peritoneal cavity. The plastic variety is the more common and the child is usually anorexic and extremely ill. The abdomen feels 'doughy' and pyrexia is usually present. The omentum is also usually affected and may be felt as an elongated tumour in the upper abdomen. Attacks of partial intestinal obstruction may occur in this type of tuberculous peritonitis.

The diagnosis of abdominal tuberculosis may be confirmed by using the Mantoux test, radiological examination, clinical examination of the chest and examining the stools for the presence of the tubercle bacillus. In cases of active tuberculosis the erythrocyte sedimentation rate (ESR) is raised.

Treatment

The treatment of abdominal tuberculosis requires rest, fresh air and an adequate diet with sufficient vitamins, together with the use of the antituberculosis drugs as mentioned previously. The prognosis in abdominal tuberculosis is worse in the younger child, and if the disease is also present in the lungs the prognosis is more serious. Cases of tabes mesenterica usually improve, but there is always the danger, especially in the early months after the primary infection, of the disease spreading by the bloodstream to produce generalised miliary tuberculosis.

Miliary tuberculosis and tuberculous meningitis (Figs 8.1 to 8.3)

Miliary tuberculosis develops when the infection has become generalised by blood-stream spread. This is a severe pyrexial condition

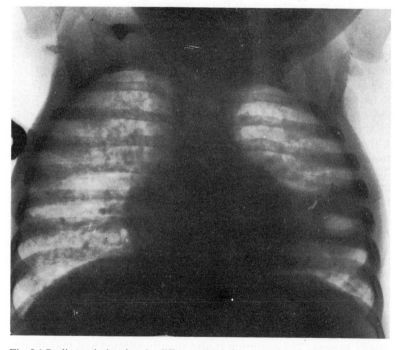

Fig. 8.1 Radiograph showing the diffuse multiple fine opacities of miliary tuberculosis affecting the lungs ('snowstorm' effect) together with a cavity in the left lung. (Infant aged 7 months.)

and the child is usually extremely ill. Evidence of the miliary infection in the lungs may be found by X-ray examination; the appearance is that of multiple small opacities spread evenly throughout the lung fields giving a 'snowstorm' effect. There is wasting, cough, and a rapid respiratory rate. Crepitations may be heard on auscultation of the lungs. This disease was always fatal, but the outlook is very much improved with the use of the antituberculosis drugs such as streptomycin, INAH and sodium PAS or the other drugs such as ethambutol or rifampicin if resistance of the organism to the usual drugs occurs.

Tuberculous meningitis. This condition develops when the blood-borne spread of the tuberculous infection involves the meninges. It is always secondary to and usually follows another tuberculous focus which has spread into the bloodstream. The onset of this disease is usually insidious, and the three symptoms which may suggest the condition are

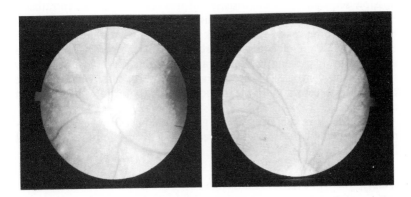

Figs 8.2 and 8.3 Choroidal tubercles seen by ophthalmological examination of the fundus of the eye in tuberculous meningitis.

headache, vomiting and constipation. The patient may become irritable and show signs of meningeal irritation, with neck stiffness and neck rigidity; squints may also develop. The child may be pyrexial and convulsions may occur. In the untreated cases this stage passes into that of the final comatose picture with eventual death. It must be stressed however that this classical description is not usually seen with the advent of modern therapy, prior to which all cases of tuberculous meningitis were fatal. The diagnosis must be confirmed by lumbar puncture and removal of cerebrospinal fluid. The pressure of the fluid is usually increased; it is clear-coloured, except that on standing a fine clot may develop. A cell count shows an increase in the number of lymphocytes with some polymorphonuclear leucocytes. The chemical investigation shows a raised protein and a lowered sugar content. To confirm the diagnosis, the tubercle bacilli should be found in a stained smear of the cerebrospinal fluid or by culture or guinea-pig inoculation.

Treatment

Good nursing is essential in the treatment of this disease and an adequate diet is most important. The drugs available, as previously stated, are isoniazid (INAH), streptomycin and PAS. Streptomycin must be given intramuscularly in the dosage mentioned and, in addition, may be administered intrathecally daily by lumbar puncture. The intrathecal dose is usually 25 mg in the small child increasing to 50 mg in the bigger child. With the introduction of INAH for the treatment of tuberculosis it is now uncommon for intrathecal therapy to be necessary, but rarely this form of treatment may still be required. PAS is given orally and INAH also by mouth. Rifampicin and ethambutol may also be used. Steroid therapy such as prednisone is also being administered to patients with tuberculous meningitis and this therapy may reduce possible sequelae from this disease but this is controversial. Intrathecal hydrocortisone is also being administered in certain cases with possible benefit. In some cases, where thick granulation tissue develops at the base of the brain blocking the circulation of the cerebrospinal fluid and thereby increasing the intracranial pressure, surgery is necessary to drain the ventricles. These therapeutic approaches, however, have become less necessary with the introduction of INAH into the treatment of this disease.

The outlook in this disease has greatly changed with modern treatment and many cases are now recovering from this formerly fatal illness.

Other forms of tuberculous infection

Cervical tuberculous adenitis. In this condition the cervical glands are affected by tuberculosis and they follow a primary tuberculous infection of the tonsils which then spreads to the draining glands. The disease is not as common as in the past, and is an insidious condition. The glands of the neck and at the angle of the jaw become enlarged and matted together. They may break down and burst through the skin producing a sinus.

Treatment requires good nursing, fresh air, a good diet and the use of the antituberculosis drugs; and also the glands may be surgically removed.

The BCG vaccine

The Bacille-Calmette-Guérin vaccine is used extensively in Scandinavia and other countries. It is an avirulent bovine strain of the tubercle bacillus and its use by intradermal injection is restricted to Mantoux negative subjects. Freeze-dried preparations of this vaccine are available. The Mantoux reaction becomes positive in about eight weeks; newborn babies and Mantoux-negative individuals, such as nurses, medical students and doctors, whose activities bring them into contact with tuberculosis, may be injected with BCG vaccine. This is to afford protection against an infection of tuberculosis. BCG vaccine is also being used as an agent to stimulate resistance to leprosy.

9. Disorders of Nutrition

In order that an individual may have optimum nutrition, not only does he require an adequate intake of the essential food elements, but digestion must be normal so that he may satisfactorily digest and then absorb and utilise these elements.

The essential food elements include protein, fat, carbohydrate, water, mineral salts and vitamins. Various deficiency diseases may develop with an absent or low intake of the different elements, and these, together with general undernutrition and malnutritional syndromes, will now be discussed.

Marasmus

This condition follows a chronic state of undernutrition. Other terms have been applied to describe this state, such as dystrophy and athrepsia or infantile atrophy. For many years there has been discussion regarding the cause of this condition. The aetiology of marasmus must include such causes as underfeeding, infection, congenital abnormalities and other conditions producing a failure to thrive. With underfeeding, the infant does not receive his calorific requirements and a condition of starvation is produced. Infection is an extremely common cause of failure to thrive, and these may be alimentary or respiratory; congenital syphilis may also give rise to this picture. Various congenital abnormalities, such as harelip, cleft-palate, pyloric stenosis, congenital heart disease, and abnormality of brain development may also be responsible. Marasmus may also affect infants born into homes of poor economic circumstances and the low birth weight infant on rare occasions passes into this state. Other important causes of a failure to thrive are coeliac disease and cystic fibrosis (fibrocystic disease of the pancreas), which have been discussed in a previous section. Gastrointestinal abnormality may also give rise to this syndrome.

Clinical features

This condition develops very slowly; the infant's weight becomes stationary and eventually the child loses weight. Any infant who has lost more than 25 per cent of his expected weight may be classified in this group. The face develops a peculiar wasted appearance and the skin becomes very lax and dry. The abdominal wall is thin and the child appears hungry. The temperature is usually below normal and

114

infection may develop, if it is not already present. Brain growth and development may be adversely affected by early undernutrition.

The treatment of the condition depends on the cause and this cause, if known, must be attacked with vigour. The diet is most important. It should commence with a skimmed milk preparation and increase slowly until the calorific intake for the child's ideal weight rather than for its actual weight is eventually reached. Careful nursing is an absolute essential in the handling of this condition, and infection should be prevented at all costs.

Malnutrition (kwashiorkor, or protein-calorie malnutrition) (Figs 9.1 to 9.5)

This disease entity affects infants in various parts of the world such as Africa, the West Indies and the Philippines. It has taken on tremendous importance and much research work has been undertaken on this problem. It is due to protein-calorie malnutrition with a low protein intake associated with a high starch diet. The clinical features include the development of oedema, irritability and depigmentation and other lesions of the skin. Hair changes occur including a tendency to become

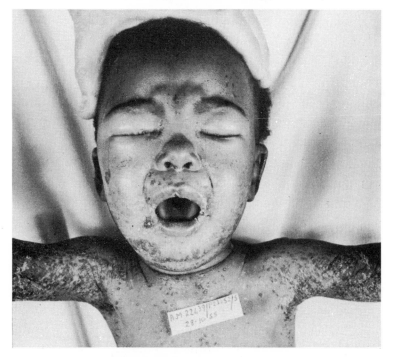

Fig. 9.1 Protein-calorie malnutrition (kwashiorkor) showing the dermatosis, oedema and angular stomatitis.

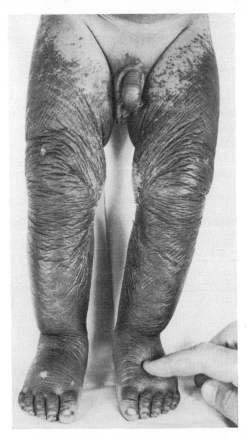

Fig. 9.2 The legs of the same patient as in previous figure showing the dermatosis and oedema.

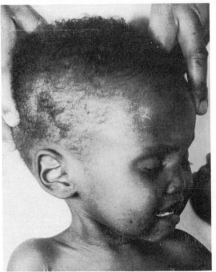

Fig. 9.3 Proteln-calorie malnutrition showing the hair changes.

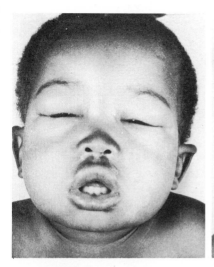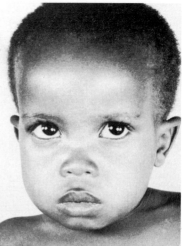

Fig. 9.4 Protein-calorie malnutrition showing oedema of the face. (Weight 9 kg. Age 1 year 9 months.)
Fig. 9.5 The same child three days later showing improvement with loss of oedema. (Weight 7·5 kg.)

lighter and also reddish in colour ('red boy'). These infants may develop diarrhoea, and their serum protein levels are reduced. They may also develop angular stomatitis.

Treatment

If treated early, these patients do well. The basis of treatment is dietetic, and the child should be given a low-fat milk preparation, supplying sufficient protein. Specific vitamin therapy plays no part in the management of this disease.

Rickets (Figs 9.6 to 9.13)

This is a deficiency disease and is associated with a low calcium condition in the body. It affects, in the usual infantile form, infants from 4 months upwards. It is due to a deficiency of vitamin D; as it is the ultraviolet light of sunshine which converts the ergosterol in the skin to vitamin D, the disease is most common in temperate countries with little sunshine and is most marked in late winter.

The clinical features of the condition mainly affects the growth of bone, and bony changes affecting different parts of the skeleton are seen. The head is affected by craniotabes, where the skull bones are softer than normal. The head appears large and may develop protuberances or bossing of the frontal and parietal areas. The ribs are affected at the costochondral junctions with the development of beading at this

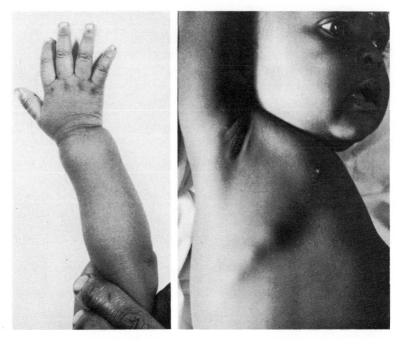

Fig. 9.6 Rickets in an infant showing the prominent ends of the radius and ulna at the wrist.
Fig. 9.7 Rickets in an infant showing the rounded swellings (beading) at the costochondral junctions of the ribs ('rickety rosary').

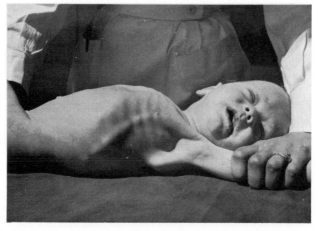

Fig. 9.8 Another infant with rickets showing a 'rickety rosary'.

area ('rickety rosary'); this beading can easily be detected by running the finger over the rib at this junction, when a rounded smooth swelling may be felt. A horizontal groove in the chest may develop, which corresponds to the pull of the diaphragm within the chest on the softened thoracic cage (Harrison's sulcus). The pelvis may be affected, producing a deformity. The extremities at the wrists and ankles are usually affected with enlargement of the epiphyses at these areas. Curvature of the bones of the extremities are easily produced by the effects of posture. These infants are hypotonic and have an associated anaemia although appearing to be well nourished; they are usually irritable and sweat profusely.

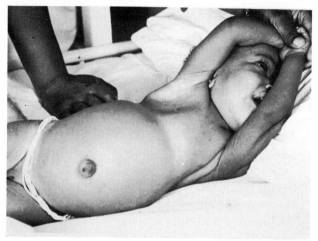

Fig. 9.9 Rickets in an infant showing Harrison's sulcus.

Examination of the blood may show a low or normal calcium and a low phosphorus content with a raised alkaline phosphatase. Radiological examination, especially of the ends of the long bones such as the radius and ulna, shows characteristic changes such as cupping, lipping, fraying and splaying of the bone-end, with osteoporosis. Rickets may be complicated by three conditions:

1. Laryngismus stridulus
2. Tetany
3. Convulsions

This triad of symptoms makes up the clinical entity of spasmophilia and is due to a low ionic calcium content of the blood, giving rise to neuromuscular irritability.

Prevention and treatment

Rickets should not occur at the present time, and in fact, with efficient community health services in the form of infant welfare centres,

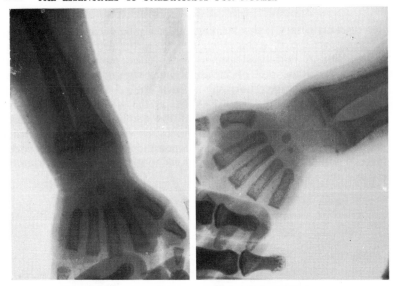

Fig. 9.10 X-ray of the wrist joint showing active florid rickets. The lower ends of the ulna and radius show the typical radiological features of cupping, splaying, fraying of the edges, lipping and osteoporosis. (Child aged 10 months.)

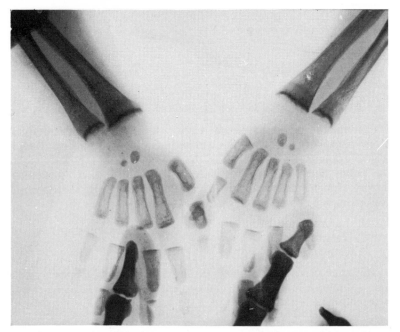

Fig. 9.11 Same case as the previous illustration showing the commencement of healing of the rickets with the laying down of calcium at the bone ends following treatment with vitamin D.

this disease is becoming more uncommon. This encouraging fact is due to the education of the public and the supply of vitamin D preparations to mothers for their infants. The normal daily requirement is about 400 i.u. of vitamin D and this amount efficiently prevents the development of a rachitic picture. In the presence of the disease, the condition may be treated by supplying vitamin D either, (1) in dosage of about 5000 units per day to these infants over a prolonged period and continuing with the normal requirement when the disease is under control, or (2) in high dosage for a limited period followed by the normal requirements.

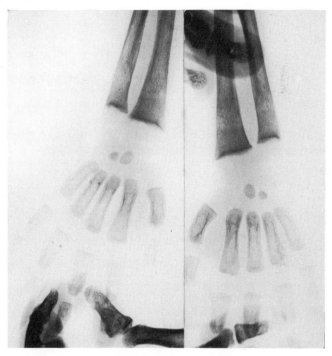

Fig. 9.12 A further stage in the healing of rickets.

Calcium need not be given if the diet is adequate and includes milk (a pint of cow's milk contains about 0·7 g of calcium). For the treatment of spasmophilia, calcium must be supplied rapidly, and the best preparation is 5 to 10 ml of intravenous 10 per cent calcium gluconate. Sunshine is also important in preventing rickets and should be used, if circumstances permit, under adequate control. Fish oils such as cod liver and halibut liver oils are a natural source of vitamin D. There are various proprietary preparations available which contain vitamin D. It should be stressed here that overdosage with this vitamin may occur with complications developing. In this connection it should be stated that most preparations containing vitamin D also contain vitamin A, and vitamin A intoxication due to overdosage also occurs. The vitamin A requirements of an infant are about 1500 to 3000 i.u. daily.

Late rickets. Rickets may affect the older child and in these cases it is usually associated with coeliac disease or chronic nephritis. In coeliac

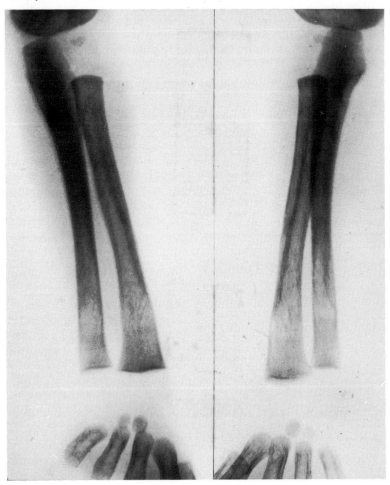

Fig. 9.13 Almost complete healing following treatment of rickets with vitamin D.

disease the rickets will not manifest itself until the child is improving from his primary condition as rickets only affects a growing bone, and bone growth will only take place in coeliac disease when it starts improving. In chronic nephritis rickets may also develop and this condition gives rise to short stature with a gross knock-knee deformity (genu valgum). This is a serious disease with a poor prognosis.

Scurvy

This disease was described many years ago by Barlow and is due to a deficiency of vitamin C (ascorbic acid). The condition manifests itself usually after the sixth month when there has been a deficiency of this vitamin. The main clinical feature in this disease is the development of subperiosteal haemorrhages affecting the long bones, usually around the elbow and knee. Blood extravasates between the periosteum and the bone and produces an extremely painful lesion; this is manifested clinically by the patient not moving the affected limb, i.e. with the development of a pseudoparalysis. Pseudoparalysis may also be caused by bone injury possibly due to child abuse, septic arthritis and osteomyelitis and also by congenital syphilis. In the latter condition, however, it usually occurs in the first six months of life. Pain is the reason for the child not moving the limb and it is therefore not a true paralysis. Other features of scurvy include spongy bleeding gums, present only if teeth have erupted, and haemorrhages around the eye. There is also anaemia and irritability; the sternum is dislocated backwards, thereby producing sharp beading at the costochondral junctions, in contrast to the smooth beading of rickets. X-ray examination of the affected limbs shows a well-marked white line of calcification near the ends of the long bones (Fraenkel's line). The subperiosteal haemorrhages may be evident on X-ray; the epiphyses have a ground-glass appearance with a sharp pencilled outline. The urine almost always contains red blood cells.

Treatment

This disease is extremely rare with proper control of infants by infant welfare centres. If it occurs, however, the treatment is to provide vitamin C which may be given in a dosage of 100 mg three times a day orally. This amount rapidly saturates the child, who should then continue with the normal daily requirement of about 50 mg. The citrus fruits such as oranges, lemons and grapefruit contain large amounts of vitamin C, and orange juice should be used in association with infant feeding. Tomato and blackcurrant juices are other sources of this vitamin. Unboiled cow's milk also contains ascorbic acid, but this is destroyed by boiling and by the pasteurisation process.

Vitamin A deficiency

Vitamin A is found in liver, butter and milk products and the carotene contained in carrots is also converted in the body to vitamin A. It is only rarely that a pure deficiency of this vitamin occurs; if it should happen, an eye condition known as xerophthalmia may develop, which if untreated may do irreparable damage to the cornea. In the older patient night blindness is an early sign of vitamin A deficiency. Three thousand units of this vitamin is the usual daily requirement for the young child, and as mentioned in a previous paragraph, intoxication due to overdosage may occur, with its effects on bone, with cortical thickening and pain. Anorexia, loss of hair and increased intracranial pressure may also occur and the serum vitamin A level is raised.

Vitamin B deficiency

The vitamin B complex is made up of various components, and pure deficiencies of some of these have been recorded. Deficiency of vitamin B_1 (thiamine, aneurine) produces the clinical picture of beri-beri. This is an oedematous condition which might be associated with polyneuritis and heart failure. The enzyme transketolase activity of the red cells is decreased. Vitamin B_2 (riboflavin) deficiency may manifest itself with angular stomatitis affecting the corners of the mouth, as discussed in a previous section. Niacin deficiency manifests itself as the disease of pellagra (Fig. 9.14). Vitamin B_6 (pyridoxine) deficiency may cause

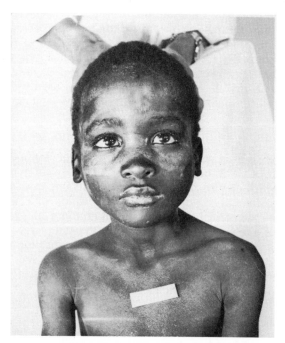

Fig. 9.14 Pellagra. This child, aged 7 years, was successfully treated with a good diet and nicotinamide.

convulsions in infancy and an inborn error of metabolism in relation to pyridoxine may also occur (pyridoxine-dependency syndrome). The treatment of all these conditions necessitates the provision of the deficient element.

10. Disorders of the Blood

The blood is made up of red and white corpuscles, platelets and plasma. At birth there is a high red cell count and haemoglobin content. There is a rapid reduction in the red cells in the first few weeks of life and a drop in the haemoglobin content in the first three months. The white cell count is slightly higher in the early years of life as compared to adults. Until the age of 4 years there is an excess of lymphocytes over the polymorphonuclear leucocytes. The platelets number approximately 250,000 per mm^3.

Anaemia

Anaemia means a reduction from the normal of the number of red blood cells or haemoglobin content, or a combination of both, i.e. a reduction in quality or quantity of the red cells. Normally there are about 5,000,000 red cells per mm^3, with a haemoglobin content of about 13·5 g per cent.

The failure of four chief mechanisms may produce anaemia:

1. Deficiency of the elements essential for normal red cell formation —dyshaemopoietic or deficiency anaemia
2. Excessive breakdown of red cells—haemolytic anaemia
3. Blood loss—haemorrhagic
4. Disease of the blood forming tissue

Dyshaemopoietic anaemia

Iron deficiency anaemia (nutritional anaemia of infancy). One of the most important deficiency anaemias of childhood is that associated with lack of iron. This is always hypochromic and microcytic (red cells being small and deficient in haemoglobin). This mechanism plays some role in the anaemia of prematurity and it occurs in the infant fed on a deficient diet. The management of iron deficiency anaemia is related more to the prevention of the condition, although once it has developed the therapy is based on supplying iron to the patient in the form of ferrous sulphate or other iron preparation. Deficiency of copper has also been postulated as a cause of this type of anaemia. Vitamin C is necessary for normal red corpuscular formation; therefore the deficiency state involving vitamin C (scurvy) is also associated with anaemia.

Thyroid secretion is also required for red cell formation so that hypo-thyroidism or cretinism may also be a cause. Folic acid deficiency may also cause anaemia (megaloblastic type.)

Infections are also important causes of anaemia in childhood, and anaemia is also found in cases of juvenile rheumatism and nephritis. Coeliac disease is often associated with a microcytic hypochromic anaemia. It has been doubtful whether true pernicious anaemia occurs in childhood but similar conditions to adult pernicious anaemia with vitamin B_{12} (cyanocobalamin) deficiency have been recorded. The treatment of the deficiency anaemias is based on supplying the deficient element. To summarise the causes of anaemia in this group, there are:

1. Nutritional anaemia of infancy or iron deficiency anaemia
2. Possible copper deficiency associated with the iron lack
3. Scurvy
4. Hypothyroidism
5. Infections
6. Rheumatism and nephritis
7. Coeliac disease
8. Folic acid deficiency

Haemolytic anaemia

This group is due to excessive destruction of the red cells; it may be caused by an antibody effect or by excessive destruction of abnormal red cells. The commonest condition of the antibody effect is erythro-blastosis foetalis in the newborn due to Rh incompatibility although this disease is being successfully prevented. Rarely, a similar condition might occur due to an ABO incompatibility, with increased production and the effects of either anti-A or anti-B antibody. In the older child, acute autoimmune haemolytic anaemia may rarely occur. It occurs rapidly with the production of an anaemia, jaundice and haemoglobinuria indicating the haemolytic nature of the condition with evidence of rapid red blood cell breakdown. It is due to circulating autoagglutinins and the Coombs test is often positive. Corticosteroid therapy is required and blood transfusion may be necessary. Haemolysis of red cells may also occur from the effects of drugs (e.g. nitrofurantoin, sulphonamides), snake bite, the fava bean (associated with an enzyme, glucose-6-phosphate dehydrogenase, deficiency) or infection. The haemolytic anaemias associated with abnormality of the red blood corpuscles are mainly:

1. Thalassaemia or Mediterranean anaemia
2. Sickle-cell disease
3. Hereditary spherocytosis or acholuric jaundice or hereditary spherocytic anaemia.

The last-mentioned condition is one of the more common of these rare diseases. Abnormal types of haemoglobin are found in some of these diseases (haemoglobinopathies).

Thalassaemia. Thalassaemia (Mediterranean anaemia or Cooley's anaemia) is a rare hereditary condition affecting people who live or originate in the Mediterranean area such as Greece, Cyprus or southern Italy and also Thailand. Some of the red cells have the microscopic appearance of targets ('target cells'). Abnormal amounts of different haemoglobin types (haemoglobin F and A_2) are found in this disease. There is an anaemia present with a leucocytosis and indications of excessive red blood cell breakdown. The spleen becomes enlarged and the patient eventually develops an extremely sallow complexion with mongoloid facies. This facial appearance is due to the thickening of the bones of the face associated with the hyperplastic marrow. The disease is progressive and the prognosis poor. Treatment requires repeated blood transfusion to maintain a haemoglobin level above 9 g per 100 ml, and the use of chelating agents such as desferrioxamine to remove excessive iron deposits. The maintenance of higher levels of haemoglobin appears to lead to improved growth with a more normal skeleton.

Sickle-cell disease. This is also a rare disease affecting the American Negro and the African. The affected red cells become sickle-shaped and the disease may present clinically with pain and swelling of the joints, enlargement of the spleen and acute haemolytic episodes. The red blood corpuscles may require special preparation in order to show the sickling manifestation. The red cells show an increased resistance to saline solutions similar to thalassaemia, but in contrast to hereditary sphero-cytic anaemia where the red cells have an increased fragility to these solutions. Sickle-cell disease is progressive with a poor prognosis. Some individuals have this trait in their blood without developing the anaemia. This disease is associated with the presence of different types of haemoglobin such as haemoglobin S and the foetal types of haemo-globin (haemoglobin F). The individuals with haemoglobin S also appear to be more resistant to malaria.

Hereditary spherocytosis (acholuric jaundice). This is a hereditary disease producing symptoms by the excessive breakdown of red blood cells. The cells show abnormality in being small and spherical in shape (microspherocytosis) and show increased fragility to saline solutions. Normally, red cells start haemolysing in saline of 0·42 per cent strength and the haemolysis is complete in saline solutions of 0·30 per cent strength (normal saline being 0·9 per cent strength). In this disease the haemolysis starts in about 0·7 per cent saline and is complete in 0·42 per cent saline, indicating increased fragility. Jaundice may occur in the neonatal period, but usually appears only in the older child. It varies in intensity, usually being very mild and disappearing entirely at times. The stools are normal in colour; the urine does not contain bile but excessive urobilin. Anaemia is present and acute haemolytic crises tend to occur. The spleen is often enlarged and there is a family history of the same disease. The treatment of the condition is to remove the spleen, and this operation cures the symptoms. It has been suggested that splenectomy in the very young may predispose to infection. The anaemia may require blood transfusion which must be given with care.

To summarise the important haemolytic anaemias, mention must be made of:

(a) Haemolytic disease of the newborn due to Rh incompatibility.
(b) Jaundice and anaemia due to isoagglutination associated with ABO incompatibility.
(c) Autoimmune haemolytic anaemia.
(d) Other haemolytic conditions due to some toxic agent such as snake bite, drugs (glucose-6-phosphate dehydrogenase deficiency) or infections.
(e) Haemolytic anaemias due to abnormality of the red cell:
  (i) Hereditary spherocytosis (acholuric jaundice)
  (ii) Thalassaemia (Mediterranean anaemia)
  (iii) Sickle-cell disease.

Haemorrhagic anaemia

This group of anaemias follows blood loss from haemorrhage, whether due to trauma or disease. The symptomatic treatment is blood replacement by transfusion if the anaemia is severe enough, and then the treatment of the basic cause.

Disease of the blood-forming tissue

This is basically the condition of *aplastic anaemia*. The bone marrow does not function adequately and there is a reduction of the red cell element of the blood in addition to a reduction of the granular white cells and the platelets. The picture of a pancytopenia is produced. There is an idiopathic type with an unknown cause. Other varieties may be due to the toxic effect on the marrow of chemical agents such as benzol, gold compounds, chloramphenicol and other drugs, or physical agents such as irradiation. A similar type may be produced by the replacement effect on the marrow of new growths or leukaemia. The child develops increasing pallor with the well-marked anaemia; haemorrhages may occur and there is no evidence of blood regeneration. The prognosis is extremely poor and blood transfusion is the only available therapy although the anabolic steroid, oxymetholone, testosterone and corticosteroid administration may be beneficial.

Leukaemia. In this disease there is a proliferation of white cells with the appearance of primitive cells in the circulation. The disease may be acute, subacute or chronic. In children it usually occurs in the acute form. It may be classified according to the type of abnormal white cell—lymphocytic, myeloid or monocytic. In children the clinical picture in all these types is similar. The cause is unknown and the age incidence in childhood, when the disease occurs most frequently, is between 4 and 8 years. It usually has a slow onset with the child developing pallor and weakness. The skin assumes a waxy appearance and pyrexia may occur. In addition, haemorrhagic manifestations make their appearance in the form of skin petechiae or mucosal bleeding. The gums may become sore and ulcerated and pains in the limbs may develop. The lymph glands become enlarged and the spleen may become palpable. A blood count shows an anaemia and a low platelet count (thrombocytopenia) with the white cell count being either high or low (aleukaemic or subleukaemic leukaemia); the white cells, however, show a high proportion of primitive types (lymphoblasts or myeloblasts). A bone marrow examination is usually essential to confirm the diagnosis of leukaemia.

The prognosis of this disease is very poor although treatment is available which does allow for remissions which may last years. The therapy that is available includes steroids (cortisone derivatives, such as prednisone), 6-mercaptopurine (Puri-Nethol), methotrexate and vincristine (Oncovin); other useful chemotherapeutic agents include L-asparaginase (Crasnitin), cytosine arabinoside (Cytosar), daunorubicin (rubidomycin, Cerubidin) and these preparations are being used with good effect in combination with each other. Many of these preparations have severe side-effects such as bone marrow depression, loss of hair and cardiotoxicity (daunorubicin). At the beginning of treatment the rapid destruction of leukaemic cells may result in an increase in the uric acid content of the blood which may give rise to kidney complications; the management of this problem is to increase the fluid intake, alkalinise the urine and administer allopurinol (Zyloric) for a few days. Cranial radiotherapy is used for prophylaxis and also for the treatment of leukaemic infiltration of the meninges. Blood transfusions may be useful as a palliative measure in the treatment of leukaemia and antibiotics are necessary to prevent infection.

Agranulocytosis. In this condition there is a gross reduction in the granular white cells (myeloid series) of the blood, associated with an ulcerative condition of the mouth and throat. The condition is most often caused by the reaction of the patient to some drug to which he is sensitive. The commonest drug to produce this condition in the past was amidopyrine; but it may also follow the use of chloramphenicol, thiouracil, sulphonamides and other drugs. Treatment requires blood transfusions and the administration of penicillin in addition to stopping the responsible drug. Corticosteroids and pyridoxine (vitamin B_6) have also been used.

The haemorrhagic diseases

In order to appreciate the bleeding diseases it is essential to be aware of the important aspects of the mechanism of the clotting of blood. The theory of coagulation or clotting is based on certain factors present in the platelets (adenosine diphosphate (ADP), 5-hydroxytryptamine, platelet factor 3) and the plasma. The platelets break down, when required for clotting, and substances interact with other substances in the plasma; plasma contains many factors which take part in clotting and these include:

(a) Antihaemophilic globulin or the antihaemophilic factor (AHG, factor VIII) which interacts with the platelet factor and with

(b) Christmas factor (plasma thromboplastin component, PTC, factor IX)

(c) Factor XI (plasma thromboplastin antecedent, PTA) and

(d) Other factors such as the Stuart-Prower factor (factor X), the Hageman factor (factor XII) and the fibrin-stabilising factor (factor XIII)

These factors interact in the first phase of the clotting mechanism to form thromboplastin (factor III) and this substance then is acted upon further by prothrombin (factor II), factor V (labile factor, proaccelerin), factor VII (stable factor, proconvertin, SPCA), together with calcium (factor IV) and other substances to form thrombin in the second phase of the clotting mechanism. Thrombin then activates the fibrinogen (factor I) of the plasma in the third phase of the clotting mechanism to form fibrin which is the basis of a clot. Other factors are also under investigation in regard to this mechanism. However, from the practical point of view the theory as outlined above allows for a classification of the conditions producing bleeding. Most of the coagulation factors are produced by the liver except factors VIII and XIII. Factor VIII (antihaemophilic factor) is probably produced by the reticuloendothelial system.

Disorders of the clotting mechanism

1. *Hypoprothrombinaemia* (low and deficient prothrombin). This condition is the basis for haemorrhagic disease of the newborn and may also follow deficiency of vitamin K intake or absorption (vitamin K is necessary for the proper synthesis of prothrombin) and liver disease (as prothrombin is formed in the liver). Vitamin K is necessary for the production of factors II, VII, IX and X.

2. *Lack of fibrinogen.* This very rarely occurs; it may do so as a congenital abnormality or be associated with liver disease. This condition may also develop during labour and produce severe postpartum haemorrhage; in these cases it may be associated with intrauterine

death of the foetus or an accidental separation of the placenta (the normal fibrinogen content of the blood is 150–400 mg per 100 ml).

3. *Haemophilia* (haemophilia A). This interesting well-known disease is due to a deficiency of antihaemophilic globulin (AHG, factor VIII) in the blood plasma. The severity of the condition depends on the degree of factor VIII deficiency. The disease is a hereditary sex-linked recessive condition affecting males only but transmitted by females, who do not themselves suffer from the disease. A female carrier of haemophilia has a 50 per cent risk of transmitting the disease to her male children and a 50 per cent risk of her female children being carriers of the condition. Excessive bleeding follows any traumatic event, even those of a trivial nature such as a simple cut or tooth extraction. The knee joints, being the most traumatised joints in little boys, are likely to become affected with swelling and pain; this is due to an effusion of blood into these joints (haemarthrosis) and if repeated they may become arthritic. Blood tests for coagulation must be done and these include the kaolin partial thromboplastin time (PTT), kaolin clotting time and the thrombotest. The bleeding time is normal and the clotting time is prolonged but this is too insensitive to be used as a screening test. The platelet count is normal and the blood shows an anaemia only if sufficient has been lost by haemorrhage.

The goal of treatment of haemophilia is the replacement of the deficient factor sufficient to stop bleeding. Direct pressure, if possible, may be useful as an immediate measure. Factor VIII, the deficient antihaemophilic globulin, is a labile substance and only present in fresh, fresh-frozen or lyophilised plasma which are administered by intravenous infusion in case of bleeding. Cryoprecipitate is used for the management of haemophilia and 1 unit per 10 kg bodyweight raises the factor VIII level by 25 per cent. Concentrates of the deficient factor, human or animal, preferably porcine, are also useful in the management of this disease, administered by intravenous infusion. If there has been much blood loss, whole blood transfusion (fresh) is essential.

4. *Christmas disease* (PTC deficiency, haemophilia B, factor IX deficiency) (Fig. 10.1). In this disease there is a deficiency of Christmas factor (factor IX, PTC) which produces a similar clinical picture to haemophilia. It also affects males and is transmitted as a sex-linked recessive condition in a similar way to true haemophilia. Christmas factor (factor IX, PTC) can be provided by administering fresh or fresh-frozen plasma in the treatment of bleeding in this disease. A concentrate containing factors II, VII, IX and X (Konyne) is available.

There are other rare conditions with bleeding as a major manifestation where the patient may have a deficiency of other constituents of plasma necessary for the clotting of blood, e.g. factor VII, factor V or factor XI deficiencies and others. Factor XI (PTA) is a labile substance and therefore is present in fresh or fresh-frozen plasma.

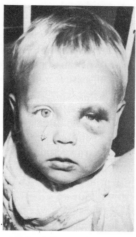

Fig. 10.1 Haematoma around the left eye of a small boy with Christmas disease (factor IX deficiency); this haematoma developed after minimal injury.

Purpura

In this condition, which is in fact a symptom, spontaneous bleeding occurs from the mucosae or into the skin or other organs. There are two large groups—thrombocytopenic (diminished platelets) and non-thrombocytopenic (normal platelets). The thrombocytopenic purpuras are made up of, firstly, a symptomatic group where the cause of the diminution of platelets is either (a) some drug such as gold, sulphona-mide or other preparation, (b) a blood disease, such as aplastic anaemia or leukaemia, or (c) some infection such as typhus fever, and secondly idiopathic thrombocytopenic purpura (ITP, essential thrombocytopenic purpura or Werlhof's disease). In this condition, for which the cause is unknown, the child bleeds spontaneously, often from the nose or into the skin or any other part. The spleen may be enlarged. The blood picture shows an anaemia, if there has been sufficient blood loss, and a lowered platelet count. The bleeding time is prolonged, but the clotting time is normal. There is an acute type, which may only have a single bleeding attack, and a chronic form which has repeated attacks. Blood transfusion of *fresh* blood or a platelet transfusion is essential to stop bleeding, and in a non-active phase of the disease in the chronic type, rarely splenectomy may be done. Corticosteroid therapy is also necessary in the treatment of this disease.

The non-thrombocytopenic purpuras are associated with normal platelets; the bleeding in this group is probably due to a defect in the capillary vessel wall. These purpuras may be due to:

1. Infections such as subacute bacterial endocarditis or meningo-coccal septicaemia

2. Drugs such as aspirin
3. Vitamin C deficiency (scurvy)
4. The mechanical effect of whooping cough or
5. The anaphylactoid purpuras (Henoch and Schönlein types)

Anaphylactoid purpura is probably due to a sensitisation of the patient by a previous streptococcal infection or other sensitising agent with the production of skin haemorrhages, mainly on the buttocks (Fig. 10.2), knees and elbows; in addition the joints may be affected (Schönlein type) or the bowel may be involved giving rise to abdominal pain with the passage of blood per rectum (Henoch's type). In these

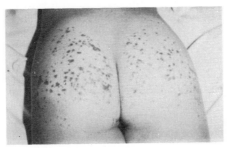

Fig. 10.2 Purpuric eruption on the buttocks in Henoch's purpura.

cases, the kidneys may also be affected, producing a similar picture to acute nephritis. Corticosteroid therapy has been tried in a number of these patients, only with slight success.

Reticuloendothelial disturbances

This system may be affected by rare conditions such as Letterer-Siwe disease, which is an acute reticulosis affecting infants and usually fatal. Lymphosarcoma also occurs rarely in childhood, affecting mainly the lymphatic glands of the chest or neck. Hodgkin's disease or lymphadenoma is another uncommon disease affecting the older child. It is a slow condition but usually progressive and affects the lymphatic glands, spleen and liver with lymphadenomatous deposits. The treatment of this disease requires radiation therapy and chemotherapy and the drugs that are used include vincristine (Oncovin), vinblastine (Velbe), nitrogen mustard (Mustine), chlorambucil (Leukeran) and cyclophosphamide (Endoxana).

Burkitt's tumour (lymphoma)

This neoplasm is the commonest type in children who live in humid, low-lying tropical areas. It usually manifests itself as a tumour of the jaws with occasional lesions in the abdominal viscera particularly the gonads and with possible invasion of the meninges. The condition is of great interest because of its geographic occurrence and also the finding of the presence of the Epstein-Barr virus (the EB virus) associated with the disease. Some of these cases have responded to chemotherapy using the cytotoxic drugs cyclophosphamide and methotrexate.

Glandular fever (infectious mononucleosis)

This disease was first recorded in 1899 by Pfeiffer. The illness has a rather uncertain incubation period from about four to seven weeks and may start acutely with a pyrexia and other constitutional symptoms. It may appear in many different forms such as with generalised enlargement of the lymph nodes mainly in the cervical region and this might be associated with a sore throat. The spleen may become palpable and enlarged and it does appear that this enlarged spleen is rather friable and injury may cause rupture. In the anginose form of infectious mononucleosis, which usually affects young adults, males more than females, the throat becomes painful and develops an exudative membrane which is whitish in appearance. This episode may persist for two weeks and does not respond to any antibiotic therapy. Various other organs may be affected including the liver with the development of hepatitis, the skin which may develop a maculopapular eruption, pinkish in colour and this rash appears readily in those patients who are given ampicillin. The disease may be prolonged in nature and may have a lengthy convalescent period. The diagnosis is supported by a positive Paul-Bunnell test indicating the presence of heterophile antibodies; these antibodies agglutinate sheep red cells and are absorbed by bovine red cells but not by guinea-pig kidney. The blood count usually shows a rise in the white cells with a large number of atypical mononuclear cells. There may be some depression of the granular cells and platelets. The immunoglobulins show a rise in the IgM and IgG levels with the IgA levels remaining unchanged. It is now established that the EB virus (EBV) is implicated in the causation of this disease. A rising titre of antibody to EB virus is found in this disease. This herpes-like virus was detected by Epstein and Barr and has been linked with other diseases such as Burkitt's tumour. There is no specific treatment for infectious mononucleosis, but bed rest, adequate nursing and symptomatic treatment are necessary. Persistent fatigue is a common complaint after infectious mononucleosis and this may persist for many months but complete recovery takes place.

Toxoplasmosis

This is a protozoal disease due to the organism *Toxoplasma gondii*. It has been mentioned previously in relation to intrauterine infection producing congenital toxoplasmosis. It may also occur as an acquired disease where it usually presents as a generalised lymphadenopathy occasionally with hepatosplenomegaly. The diagnosis may be confirmed by the complement fixation test and the Sabin-Feldman dye test. This disease may respond to the administration of pyrimethamine (Dara-prim) and the sulphonamides such as sulphadiazine. Spiramycin (Rovamycin) may also be useful.

Chronic granulomatous disease of childhood

This is a rare serious clinical syndrome usually affecting young male children and having a familial tendency. It appears to be mainly trans-mitted on a hereditary basis as a sex-linked condition (linked to the X chromosome). In this disease the main clinical features are recurrent suppurative and granulomatous lesions affecting the lymph glands, lung, skin, liver and bones. The suppurative lesions are usually due to organisms of low virulence such as certain strains of staphylococci and also Gram-negative organisms but usually not the streptococcus. The response to these infections is to produce chronic granulomatous changes. The immunoglobulins in these patients are normal but changes have been found in the polymorphonuclear neutrophils in the peripheral blood in that they show a defect with lessened bactericidal activity against staphylococci and Gram-negative organisms. Treatment requires the surgical drainage of suppurative lesions and the use of bactericidal antibiotics in high dosage.

11. Juvenile Rheumatism

Rheumatic fever has become less common and Sydenham's rheumatic chorea (St Vitus' Dance) even more uncommon. Both conditions may affect the heart, and it is this complication of rheumatic carditis which makes the disease so serious.

Rheumatic fever

This disease affects children most commonly between the ages of 5 and 10 years; it is extremely uncommon under the age of 3, and rare from 3 to 5. It is probably due to a sensitisation reaction of the patient's tissues to a previous Lancefield group A β-haemolytic streptococcal infection. This sensitisation produces a tissue reaction in which Aschoff's nodes are seen microscopically to be made up of giant cells and fibroblasts. This lesion is present in the affected parts such as the heart but not in the brain. The disease has been found more commonly in damp surroundings and among people of poorer circumstances; however, it is also found in all sections of the population in different parts of the world.

The clinical features are such that the patient usually gives a history of having had a sore throat (haemolytic streptococcal) about 10 to 20 days before the onset of the rheumatic fever. Sweating occurs and the patient may be pyrexial with a rapid pulse. There is pain in the affected joints and these may be flitting in nature, passing from joint to joint. On occasions the affected joints are reddened and swollen, but this type of presentation is uncommon. The joints most commonly affected are the knees, wrists, elbows and ankles. They may be extremely painful, and usually more than one joint is affected.

The most feared complication is that of rheumatic carditis where the heart is affected; this condition will be discussed in another section. Carditis occurs in a large proportion of cases of rheumatic fever and the treatment of this disease is aimed at preventing or alleviating this complication.

In 1944 T. D. Jones* suggested that certain clinical features should be present to substantiate a diagnosis of juvenile rheumatism; these suggestions were modified in 1965 by a Committee of the American Heart Association† which suggested that the clinical manifestations

* *Journal of the American Medical Association*, vol. 126, p. 481.
† *Circulation*, vol. 32, p. 664.

could be divided into major and minor features. The major features are carditis, polyarthritis, chorea, subcutaneous nodules and erythema marginatum (Fig. 11.1) and the minor features being fever, arthralgia, prolonged PR interval in the electrocardiogram, increased erythrocyte sedimentation rate, a rise in the antistreptolysin O titre (ASO), a family history of rheumatic fever, presence of C-reactive protein in the blood, leucocytosis, evidence of a preceding β-haemolytic streptococcal infection, a previous history of rheumatic fever and the presence of inactive rheumatic disease. It has been suggested that the presence of two major manifestations or one major and two minor manifestations supports the diagnosis of rheumatic fever, although it is not wise to be too rigid in entirely accepting this approach to the diagnosis of this disease.

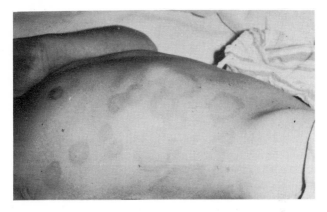

Fig. 11.1 Erythema marginatum as seen in rheumatic fever.

Treatment

The child should have bed rest in the acute phase. Careful nursing is essential in this phase and the diet must be light with adequate fluids. Salicylate in the form of buffered aspirin can be used. Rheumatic fever symptoms respond dramatically to salicylate therapy, with a reduction in temperature and the rapid disappearance of the joint pains; it may be said that if the joint pains are not better after 48 hours of adequate salicylate therapy, the disease is not rheumatic fever. Unfortunately, salicylate therapy has no effect in preventing or improving the cardiac complications of this disease. Bed rest should be prolonged for anything up to six weeks and even longer if the heart is affected, when the activity of the disease will determine the progress of the treatment. An essential therapeutic need in this disease is for an antistreptococcal drug, and for this purpose penicillin is the best agent to use. It is necessary to continue penicillin therapy for an extremely prolonged period, long after the acute phase of the disease has passed. This need cannot be sufficiently stressed as it is definitely clear that the recurrence rate of rheumatic fever has been drastically reduced with the prolonged prophylactic use of penicillin.

The steroids (cortisone or its derivatives such as prednisone or prednisolone) have been used in treating rheumatism, alone or in combination with salicylates, and there is no doubt that the general condition of the child is rapidly improved; there is, however, disappointment in the effect of these preparations in preventing cardiac complications. The convalescence must be very gradual, and careful note must be made of any signs of reactivation of the disease.

Sydenham's chorea (St Vitus' dance)

This condition is rare and has been called rheumatism of the brain. It affects females more commonly than males, and the commonest age incidence is between 5 and 10 years. The type of child affected is usually bright and intelligent and the first manifestation of the disease may be that the child starts dropping her eating utensils at table. Or, she may become fidgety at school, and it may be difficult for the teacher to recognise that this is not naughtiness, but the onset of an illness. Subsequent to this onset, the symptomatology is made up of three main features:

1. *Choreiform movements.* These are involuntary, purposeless, non-repetitive movements and may affect any part of the child, usually the limbs. The face may be affected when the child produces various contortions of the facial muscles.
2. *Inco-ordinated voluntary movements.* The voluntary movements of these patients are very inco-ordinate, and if the child is asked to perform some simple movement such as unbuttoning her pyjama jacket she may find this impossible in the acute phase of the disease or only perform it with extreme difficulty. When the child starts improving, an excellent bedside clinical test of the co-ordination of voluntary movement is to ask her to write her name, repeating the process at intervals to show the improvement in the handwriting; in the acute phase the patient finds writing impossible.
3. *Emotional instability.* These patients are very emotional and are easily upset by the least disturbance.

Other signs are found in this disease such as the snake-like movement of the tongue on protrusion and retraction. On firmly clasping a patient's hand, the alternate contraction and relaxation of the muscles are felt. The reflexes such as the knee jerks vary in this disease from absence to exaggeration of the responses and occasionally the 'hung up' type of response.

There are different varieties of chorea:

(a) The usual form which has been described

(b) The rare paralytic form where the child appears to be completely flaccidly paralysed; with careful observation, minor choreiform movements of the fingers and thumb can be observed

(c) The maniacal type of chorea, where the patient has extremely violent movements which may lead to injury if sufficient protection is not provided. In rare cases speech may be temporarily lost, but this always returns with improvement.

The disease tends to recur and the patient may have second or third attacks. The main complication is rheumatic carditis, which, if it occurs, will do so most commonly in the first attack. Carditis appears to affect approximately one out of every four or five patients during the first attack of chorea. If it does not occur in the first attack, there is a much lesser chance of it happening in the second and subsequent attacks.

Chorea must be differentiated from habit spasms or tics. These, however, are always repetitive movements, usually of a single type, whereas choreiform movements are non-repetitive and multiple.

Treatment

The basic treatment of this condition is bed rest; there is no specific drug which will cure the disease. The usual duration of the disease is about six weeks upwards, and it should be stressed that the prognosis for the choreiform movements itself is always good. The drugs to be used in chorea are the sedatives, and such preparations as phenobarbitone or some other sedative in appropriate dosage should be prescribed; chlorpromazine or the tranquillisers, such as hydroxyzine (Atarax) or meprobamate (Equanil, Miltown) may also be useful in the treatment of this disease. Careful nursing is essential in the acute phase and the child must take an adequate light diet. Corticosteroid therapy has also been used but is of no value in chorea itself. It is interesting to observe that cases of rheumatic fever may subsequently develop attacks of chorea and vice versa.

Rheumatoid arthritis (Fig. 11.2)

In this disease there is a periarticular inflammatory reaction of various joints. Males are affected as frequently as females in childhood and the disease usually starts over the age of 3 years. The onset may be slow or rapid. If it is rapid, there may be pyrexia and swelling of joints. The knees, wrists, elbows, ankles and spine may be affected and frequently the small joints of the fingers are also involved. The joints become swollen and tender and the corresponding muscles become wasted. There is frequently an associated lymphatic reaction in these patients, with enlargement of the lymphatic glands and the spleen. When this combination occurs, the name of Still's disease is given to this condition in childhood. There is frequently an associated anaemia and the erythrocyte sedimentation rate (ESR) is raised when the disease is active. Tests for the rheumatoid factor may be useful, such as the Rose-Waaler or the Latex fixation tests. On rare occasions the condition may be complicated by pericardial affection of the heart (pericarditis). This condition is very chronic and periods of remission occur.

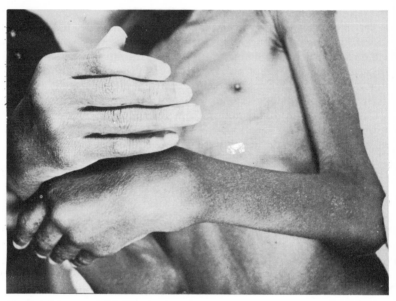

Fig. 11.2 Rheumatoid arthritis.

Treatment

In treating this disease, any septic focus must be treated and bed rest is required in the active phase. General nursing care is essential and the patient must receive an adequate diet with sufficient vitamins. A physiotherapist should co-operate in the treatment with active and passive movements and the appropriate use of splints to prevent deformities of the limbs. Aspirin may be useful. In past years, gold preparations by injection were used as treatment. The corticosteroids are another form of therapy for this disease and in appropriate cases their use is beneficial as may also be the drugs indomethacin (Indocid), benorylate (Benoral), and ibuprofen (Brufen).

12. Disorders of the Cardiovascular System

The main disorders of the cardiovascular system are those that affect the heart and great vessels. They may be affected by congenital or acquired conditions; the main acquired disease of the heart during childhood is rheumatic carditis and its sequelae.

Congenital heart disease (congenital morbus cordis)

The development of the heart in the embryo may be detrimentally affected at different stages, with the production of different anatomic defects in the heart structure; these defects may give rise to abnormality in the circulation of the blood. The normal circulation after birth allows for the passage of arterial oxygenated blood from the left ventricle via the aorta to the body; this blood gives up its oxygen and returns as venous blood via the superior and inferior venae cavae to the right auricle. It then passes through the tricuspid opening to the right ventricle and then via the pulmonary arteries to the lungs for oxygenation; oxygenated blood returns from the lungs via the pulmonary veins to the left auricle, and then flows via the mitral opening to the left ventricle for its onward pumping through the aorta as before.

Great attention has been focused on the possible causation of these heart defects, and much stimulation was given to this research by the discovery in 1941 by Gregg in Australia of the association of rubella infection occurring in a pregnant woman in the early weeks of her pregnancy and the development of congenital abnormality (including congenital heart disease) in the foetus. Certain other congenital abnormalities (Fig. 12.1) such as Down's syndrome (mongolism) and the very rare abnormality of arachnodactyly (spider fingers with eye abnormalities—Marfan's syndrome) are frequently associated with congenital heart disease.

Congenital abnormality of the heart and great vessels may or may not allow for abnormal mixture of arterial and venous blood in abnormal situations (shunt of blood). If there is a shunt of blood from the venous to the arterial side (right side to left) then cyanosis will result; if there is a left to right shunt or no shunt of blood, then cyanosis does not occur. A clinical classification of congenital heart disease can therefore be offered in relation to the presence or absence of cyanosis, and this

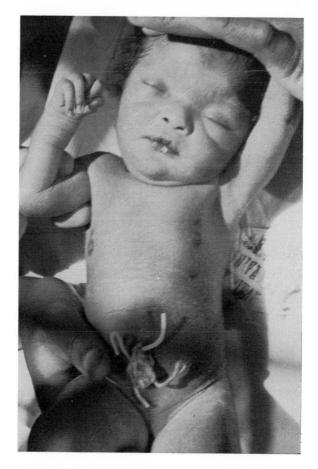

Fig. 12.1 Newborn child with supernumerary nipples. This infant also had the congenital heart abnormality of Fallot's tetralogy. (*By courtesy from Kessel: 'British Medical Journal'.*)

clinical classification can be related to abnormality of blood circulation (haemodynamics):

1. Non-cyanotic types
     (a) Never cyanosed (no shunt)
     (b) Not cyanosed, but may theoretically become cyanosed (left to right shunt; may become cyanosed if this shunt is reversed)
2. Cyanotic types (right to left shunt)

The important clinical conditions in these groups must be mentioned:

1. (a) Non-cyanotic: never cyanosed
        Dextrocardia
        Coarctation of the aorta
        Subaortic stenosis
        Abnormalities of the great vessels
   (b) Non-cyanotic but potentially cyanosed
        Patent ductus arteriosus
        Atrial septal defect
        Ventricular septal defect
2. Cyanotic ('blue baby')
        Fallot's tetralogy
        Atrial septal defect with pulmonary stenosis
        Tricuspid atresia
        Transposition of the great vessels.

There are other more rare congenital abnormalities of the heart, but they may all be placed in their respective groups.

Dextrocardia. In this condition the heart is found on the right side of the chest rather than its normal position on the left. It may be associated with complete transposition of all the thoracic and abdominal organs (*situs inversus*) (Fig. 12.2). In this type of dextrocardia the heart is usually completely normal, and the condition may be diagnosed by clinical examination. X-ray examination of the chest will confirm the abnormal position of the heart. Another type of dextrocardia, where it is present as an isolated abnormality without situs inversus of the other organs, is usually associated with some other abnormality of the heart itself, and this of necessity gives the condition a much worse prognosis than the first type.

Coarctation of the aorta. This is an uncommon abnormality which is found more frequently in males than females. In this condition there is a narrowing or stenosis of the aorta distal to the origin of the great vessels to the upper extremity and head. In view of the obstruction to the arterial flow, a collateral circulation develops in an attempt to get blood to that part of the body below the obstruction in the aorta. Clinically this condition may be diagnosed by the absence of the femoral pulses and by finding hypertension in the upper limbs and a low blood pressure in the legs. There may be clinical evidence of the collateral circulation; radiology and electrocardiography are useful in confirming the diagnosis. This condition is amenable to treatment by surgery as will be discussed later. It has been recognised that a coarctation of the aorta may present in early infancy with acute symptoms of cardiac failure. In these cases, it is necessary to control the cardiac failure and repair the abnormality surgically but even with this approach the mortality from this condition in this age-group is high.

Abnormalities of the great vessels. Various rare anomalies of the aortic arch and great vessels may occur. These abnormalities may

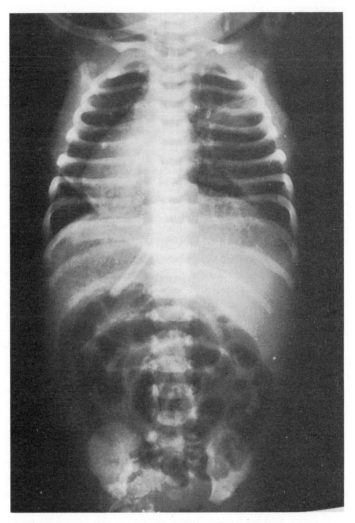

Fig. 12.2 X-ray of a newborn child with dextrocardia and situs inversus.

produce symptoms of difficulty in swallowing or breathing by pressure on the trachea and oesophagus; if sufficiently severe, surgical measures may be adopted to relieve the pressure.

Patent ductus arteriosus. This abnormality occurs more often in females and is important to diagnose as it may be cured by surgery. In this condition the foetal ductus arteriosus joining the aorta to the pulmonary artery remains patent after birth. Cyanosis does not occur except occasionally as a terminal event. These patients do not thrive well; on clinical examination an important sign is the typical 'machinery'

(Gibson) murmur heard at the pulmonary area of the praecordium. There are other important features in the symptomatology; radiology and electrocardiography are necessary confirmatory investigations. The danger of subacute bacterial endocarditis developing in this condition will be discussed later in addition to a discussion of the therapy of this abnormality. In infancy a patent ductus arteriosus may produce cardiac failure and this fact must be borne in mind as it is necessary in such cases to surgically repair the abnormality after the cardiac failure has been controlled.

Atrial septal defect. In this condition there is a defect in the septum between the two auricles of the heart with an abnormal pumping of blood from the left side to the right. This gives rise to an increased blood flow through the lungs with enlargement of the right side of the heart, and its sequelae. Radiology and electrocardiography are necessary in the diagnosis. When a pulmonary stenosis is present as an additional anomaly the shunt of blood through the atrial septal defect may be reversed from right to left with the development of cyanosis in the patient.

Ventricular septal defect. In this abnormality there is a defect in the septum between the ventricles allowing an abnormal mixture of blood from left side to right. If the shunt is small, there may not be much disability (Maladie de Roger), but with a large shunt of blood certain sequelae may occur; there is always the danger of subacute bacterial endocarditis developing in this condition. This lesion may close spontaneously.

Fallot's tetralogy. This is the commonest cause of cyanotic congenital heart disease (Fig. 12.3) and is important to diagnose as it is amenable

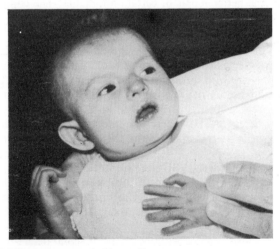

Fig. 12.3 Cyanotic congenital heart disease.

to surgery as will be discussed later. The tetralogy is made up of four anomalies of the heart; these are a pulmonary stenosis, a high ventricular septal defect with a dextroposed aorta overriding this defect and thus receiving blood both from right and left ventricles, and an enlarged right ventricle. These patients are cyanotic from birth or later, and become dyspnoeic and distressed with any exertion. They often take on a characteristic squatting posture when resting. Clubbing of the fingers occurs and the clinical features include various signs found on examination, with characteristic X-ray findings ('boot-shaped' heart) and electrocardiogram.

Treatment

In relation to the modern trends of cardiac surgery and the importance of correct diagnosis of congenital heart disease, various methods of investigation have been developed. These methods include cardiac catheterisation, to detect anomalies of pressures and oxygen concentrations in the heart and great vessels, and angiocardiography and cine-angiocardiography to show abnormalities of the heart and vessels by using radio-opaque media and X-rays. Differential dye studies are also being used in these investigations.

Congenital heart disease is an important part of cardiology and treatment is available for many different types. At one time very little beyond symptomatic measures could be done for these unfortunate patients. However, with the tremendous strides made in thoracic and cardiac surgery, many of these cases can be alleviated or cured by surgical measures. The use of a heart–lung machine to oxygenate the blood of a patient and bypass the cardiac circulation has allowed for the treatment of many hitherto untreatable abnormalities and furthermore allows for the better repair of certain anomalies. The conditions which may be treated by surgery include the following:

1. Patent ductus arteriosus (PDA), when the ductus is ligated.
2. Coarctation of the aorta, where the stenosed segment of aorta may be surgically resected and the normal ends of the vessels anastomosed, if necessary with the use of an arterial or artificial graft; this is a difficult operation, but is being undertaken in cardiac surgical clinics with great success.
3. Atrial septal defect (ASD), where the defect is now being successfully closed; if large, this may require the insertion of an artificial graft.
4. Ventricular septal defect (VSD), where again the defect is being closed successfully, with the use of the by-pass method with the heart–lung oxygenator equipment. The operation of banding the pulmonary artery is an additional procedure sometimes performed on these patients.
5. Pulmonary stenosis with or without an atrial septal defect may be relieved by the Brock operation of pulmonary valvotomy.

6. Fallot's tetralogy, which may in certain cases be anatomically repaired with the use of the by-pass method; where this is not possible the condition may be alleviated by allowing more blood to flow to the lungs by anastomosing the systemic to the pulmonary circulation (Blalock-Taussig operation of anastomosing the subclavian to the pulmonary artery or the Waterston shunt of anastomosing the ascending aorta to the right pulmonary artery or other modification) and thereby producing an artificial ductus arteriosus. The Brock procedure of pulmonary valvotomy has also been performed on this type of case to increase the blood flow to the lungs.

7. Aortic or subaortic stenosis is also being successfully treated by the cardiac surgeon.

8. Abnormalities of the aorta, e.g. a double aortic arch with its compression effects on neighbouring structures such as the trachea and oesophagus, where the smaller part of the arch may be divided to relieve the pressure.

9. Transposition of the great vessels is being treated surgically by creating a defect in the atrial septum with the Rashkind balloon technique using the foramen ovale (atrial septostomy). A further corrective procedure for this condition is the Mustard operation which alters and tends to correct the flow of blood.

10. Tricuspid atresia is being operated on with a view to increasing the pulmonary blood flow; the Glenn operation is one of the procedures being performed (anastomosis of the superior vena cava to the pulmonary artery). Arterial anastomoses such as the Blalock-Taussig operation is also used.

Prolonged discussion has taken place regarding heart transplantation since the original operation performed by Barnard, but this has been particularly applicable to adult patients with fatal cardiac conditions and has no place in paediatric cardiology.

Great interest is being shown in serious congenital heart disease in the newborn. These cases may present as congestive cardiac failure or cyanosis in the early or late neonatal period. The infants with congestive cardiac failure may have coarctation of the aorta with associated defects, a hypoplastic or atretic aorta or endocardial fibroelastosis as a cause. The cyanotic infants may be associated with transposition of the great vessels, Fallot's tetralogy or total anomalous pulmonary venous return as possible causes. Careful assessment of newborn infants in relation to the possibility of severe congenital cardiac abnormalities being present is essential in order that early precise diagnosis with subsequent treatment can be offered in order to reduce the high mortality.

All cases of congenital heart disease, except that of an atrial septal defect, are liable to develop infection at the abnormal site producing bacterial endocarditis. This is an extremely serious disease and it may also complicate cases of rheumatic heart disease; the causative organism is the *Streptococcus viridans*, which produces vegetations at the affected sites, but other organisms such as *Staphylococcus aureus* or *Escherichia coli* may also be responsible. These patients have a pyrexia, tachycardia, toxaemia, signs of embolic phenomena such as petechial haemorrhages, splinter haemorrhages under the nails, clubbing of the fingers, cerebral embolic phenomena, splenomegaly and red cells in the urine. The diagnosis may be confirmed by finding the causative organism in blood cultures. Fortunately, with the availability of antibiotics this previously fatal disease can now be adequately treated. It requires prolonged antibiotic therapy to overcome this disease. As a prophylactic measure against subacute bacterial endocarditis developing in susceptible patients with congenital or rheumatic heart disease following minor operations like tonsillectomy or tooth extractions, penicillin should be given before and after such procedures.

Rheumatic heart disease

Rheumatic carditis is the commonest acquired affection of the heart in childhood and it may complicate all cases of juvenile rheumatism such as rheumatic fever and Sydenham's chorea. As discussed in a previous section, the aetiology of the condition is related to a sensitisation reaction of the patient to a previous Lancefield group A β-haemolytic streptococcal infection (usually of the throat) occurring about 14 days before the rheumatic manifestations occur. The symptomatology of the carditis may be associated with evidence of rheumatic fever, chorea or rheumatic nodules. Carditis is manifested by signs of heart involvement with activity of the rheumatism; these signs include tachycardia, cardiac enlargement, murmurs which alter at different stages of the disease, raised sedimentation rate and raised antistreptolysin O titre, C-reactive protein, anaemia and electrocardiographic changes. Cardiac failure may occur during the acute attack or as a sequel to chronic affection of the heart. Pericarditis may also occur in these cases and, if severe, the outlook is poor. Juvenile rheumatism is very likely to relapse with the occurrence of repeated attacks. The prognosis of carditis depends on whether permanent heart damage has occurred; it should be remembered that these patients with rheumatic carditis may recover completely.

Treatment

Treatment requires bed rest until all signs of activity have disappeared. These signs include the pulse rate (the sleeping pulse rate should always be taken and used as an indication of the true rate), clinical progress and raised sedimentation rate. Other therapeutic procedures include the administration of penicillin, salicylates as aspirin and corticosteroid therapy. The last-mentioned is useful to increase general clinical improvement, but does not appear to have any dramatic effect in preventing cardiac damage. Digoxin is useful in cases of cardiac failure. The prevention of relapses is important and this is related to preventing haemolytic streptococcal infections. A necessary prophylactic measure in rheumatic subjects is to institute the routine regular daily administration of oral penicillin or small dosage sulphadiazine in penicillin-sensitive individuals over a prolonged period measured in years.

The commonest chronic disease of the heart caused by rheumatism is mitral stenosis with or without aortic incompetence. These conditions take some years to develop and the clinical picture is similar to that in the adult patient. The disease may be complicated by cardiac failure or bacterial endocarditis. Surgical treatment of mitral stenosis by valvotomy has been developed with success; this operation, however, is not often performed in childhood because the danger of reactivation of the rheumatic disease is present in this age-group. Valve replacement surgery is available as a method of treatment for the severely damaged valve in the adult patient.

Cardiac failure

Cardiac failure may occur in rheumatic heart disease, diphtheritic myocarditis, congenital heart disease and other rare cardiac conditions. Failure of the heart is shown clinically by the same signs as in the adult patient, with breathlessness, cyanosis, enlarged heart, dilated neck veins, and an enlarged tender liver with oedema. The treatment requires expert nursing, bed rest, oxygen, digoxin and diuretics such as chlorothiazide or frusemide (Lasix).

Diphtheria may be complicated on rare occasions by myocarditis which is an extremely serious condition. It usually occurs towards the end of the second week of the illness and gives rise to cardiac dilatation; sudden death may occur with the least exertion on the part of the patient. The electrocardiogram confirms the diagnosis. Absolute bed rest is essential, together with the most careful nursing.

Uncommon abnormalities of heart rhythm may occur in infancy and childhood. These include such conditions as paroxysmal tachycardia and heart block. The former, if allowed to continue uncontrolled, may lead to cardiac failure; these cases in infancy are usually well controlled by digitalisation. Certain beta-adrenergic blocking drugs are available for the treatment of some cardiac arrhythmias; these drugs include propanolol (Inderal) where the oral dose is 0·5 to 1 mg per kg bodyweight daily in three to four doses, and related preparations such as oxprenolol (Trasicor). Where rapid conversion of an arrhythmia to sinus rhythm is needed cardioversion (electrical conversion) is valuable. This requires the delivery of a synchronised impulse by a direct current machine.

13. Disorders of Metabolism

There are numerous disorders of metabolism which affect children, some common and others extremely rare (Figs 13.1 and 13.2).

Obesity

The fat child is frequently brought by the parents for medical advice. This type of child is found more commonly in the older age-group. Physiologically, the regulation of weight gain is based on the food intake in relation to the energy requirements of the individual. The commonest cause of obesity in childhood is overeating, mainly of carbohydrates;

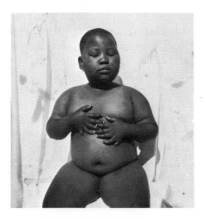

Fig. 13.1 Child, aged 5½ years, showing obesity and polydactyly (rare disease of the Laurence-Moon-Biedl syndrome).

in addition, in some such patients there is a psychological cause present in relation to hypothalamic function. Endocrine causes of obesity are extremely rare, but these must be excluded when dealing with any case of an overweight child; the endocrine glands at fault may be the suprarenals or the thyroid gland. Fröhlich's syndrome is a rare cause of obesity and is related to the small 'fat boy' type of patient who is always undersized but obese with sexual underdevelopment.

150

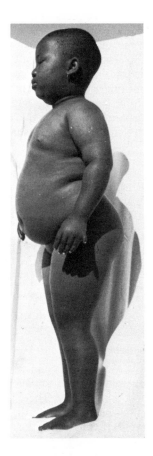

Fig. 13.2 A lateral view of the same child. (*By courtesy from Kessel: 'Journal of Pediatrics'*.)

Diabetes mellitus

This disease occurs in childhood and often presents itself as an acute illness with the child in coma or incipient coma. Initially, the symptoms are usually thirst, polyuria and tiredness. The diagnosis may be made by an examination of the urine for the presence of sugar (glucose) and acetone. This may be confirmed by finding a high fasting blood sugar level (normal 3·5–5·5 mmol per litre).

In treating cases of diabetes mellitus in children insulin is always required, and in addition the dietetic control is important as the child requires a sufficient diet to allow for adequate growth. A useful dietetic guide is to allow the child about 1000 calories plus 100 calories for each year of life per day (e.g. a child of 6 years will require a daily diet of 1600 calories); this diet may be made up of carbohydrate, protein and fat in a ratio of about $2\frac{1}{2}:1:1$. Some authorities favour an unrestricted diet except for some control of excessive carbohydrate, but a fairly restricted controlled diet is preferable. The insulin requirements should be calculated with the patient under a fair amount of control, and a start should be made with soluble insulin at the outset of treatment; later, the long-acting insulin preparations such as the insulin zinc suspensions (IZS, lente, semilente, ultralente), isophane insulin (NPH) or protamine

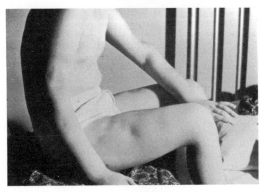

Fig. 13.3 Insulin atrophy in a diabetic patient.

zinc insulin (PZI) may be used in order to control the disease with the minimum number of injections per day. There is always the danger of an excessive insulin effect on the patient with the reduction of the blood sugar to dangerous levels (hypoglycaemia). This phase produces symptoms such as headache, irritability, pallor, sweating, trembling and occasionally convulsions and coma; they should be avoided by reducing the insulin requirements and immediately giving the child sugar (which should always be carried by all diabetics for emergency use). A preparation, glucagon, is available for use in treating hypoglycaemia. It is administered by subcutaneous, intramuscular or intravenous injection; glucagon is the secretion of the alpha cells of the islets of Langerhans whereas insulin is the secretion produced by the beta cells.

Diabetic coma. This is the most serious complication of diabetes. The patient often has abdominal pain, constipation and a dry skin with a rapid pulse rate. The breath smells of acetone and the breathing is rapid with the typical wide excursion of air hunger; coma rapidly supervenes. The urine contains much sugar, acetone and diacetic acid. Urgent therapy is essential to save life and this includes intravenous fluid therapy to correct dehydration and electrolytic dysbalance, and the provision of sufficiently large amounts of soluble insulin. The urine must be tested at frequent intervals, being obtained by catheterisation, if necessary. Blood sugar estimations should be done for effective control of treatment.

Cyclical vomiting

This type of vomiting has been discussed in a previous chapter.

Diabetes insipidus

This condition is completely different from diabetes mellitus and will be discussed later.

Inborn errors of metabolism

These are a very rare group of diseases and may affect different aspects of metabolism. One group affects lipoid metabolism and gives rise to the following diseases:

1. Gaucher's disease, in which abnormal deposits of glucocerebroside occur in different parts of the body. These patients have a greatly enlarged spleen with an enlarged liver (Fig. 13.4), and have deposits in bones such as the femur. The condition is progressive and there is no known specific treatment.
2. Niemann-Pick disease, which is a condition affecting young infants, is fatal in about 18 months and having abnormal deposits of a phospholipid sphingomyelin. Hepatosplenomegaly is present and the central nervous system is involved. It is related in some way to the fatal degenerative nervous system disease of amaurotic family idiocy (Tay-Sachs disease, infantile form of cerebromacular degeneration) which affects mainly the Jewish race. The diagnosis is confirmed by finding the typical 'cherry-red' spot at the macula of the eye by ophthalmoscopic examination.
3. Hand-Schüller-Christian disease, with its abnormal deposits of cholesterol and cholesterol esters in such areas as the cranial bones, the hypothalamus, the orbit, the lungs and the skin. Deep X-ray therapy may improve these cases and the corticosteroids may be helpful, but there is no specific therapy available.

Another rare metabolic condition related to carbohydrate metabolism is glycogen storage disease where abnormal amounts of glycogen occur in the liver, heart or kidneys. Different types of this disorder occur related to different enzyme defects and these include Von Gierke's disease in which the liver is greatly enlarged. Another type is Pompe's disease in which the glycogen deposits occur in cardiac muscle, tongue and muscles. The glycogen is not converted to glucose giving rise to a low blood sugar and ketone bodies (acetone) in the urine.

Other rare metabolic disorders include two conditions which may present clinically in infancy as a failure to thrive with vomiting and constipation. These diseases are renal acidosis of infancy and idiopathic hypercalcaemia, both of which Lightwood and his colleagues have described. The former condition is usually associated with the infant passing a persistently alkaline urine whilst in a state of acidosis; treatment is effective using alkalising salts (e.g. sodium citrate and

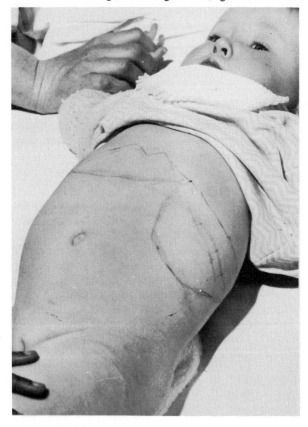

Fig. 13.4 Infant with hepatosplenomegaly due to a reticulosis storage condition similar to Gaucher's disease.

citric acid). It has become exceedingly rare. Idiopathic hypercalcaemia in infancy has similar clinical features to renal acidosis but these cases have a raised serum calcium and plasma protein level. This disease occurs in a mild and severe form; in the latter type the child may have an 'elfin facies' and be mentally subnormal and may also have cardiovascular lesions such as aortic stenosis of the supravalvular type or pulmonary artery stenosis. A low calcium diet (Locasol) is necessary in the management of this disease and corticosteroid therapy might be useful.

Another rare metabolic disorder is the Lesch-Nyhan syndrome; this is inherited as an X-linked condition. In this disease there is an enzyme deficiency (similar to that found in gout) which leads to an error of purine metabolism giving rise to raised levels of uric acid in the blood (normal blood levels of uric acid are 120–340 umol per litre). The clinical features of this syndrome include mental retardation, choreoathetoid movements and self-mutilation.

Galactosaemia. This condition is associated with the inability of the individual to properly metabolise lactose resulting in galactose accumulation. This inability is due to the absence of the enzyme galactose-1-phosphate uridyl transferase and is inherited as an autosomal recessive condition. The enzyme is necessary for normal lactose metabolism and various serious symptoms might result from the accumulation of galactose. These symptoms include a failure to thrive, vomiting, jaundice with liver involvement, cataracts in the lens of the eyes and mental defect. The diagnosis may be made by finding galactose in the urine; this type of sugar is a reducing agent and can be detected in the urine by the usual tests for reducing substances (Clinitest) after which confirmation is sought by identifying the reducing agent by chromatography. The enzyme defect may be found in the red blood cells. The management of this disease requires that lactose in all forms must be completely excluded from the diet; this of necessity requires that milk or milk products containing lactose must be prohibited to these patients. Various milk substitutes are available for the feeding of such infants (Galactomin).

Phenylketonuria (PKU). This rare condition is associated with severe mental subnormality and is transmitted as an autosomal recessive hereditary disease. It is mainly seen in fair-haired, fair-skinned children with blue eyes and infantile eczema may be an associated feature. They also tend to have a musty odour. The disorder is due to the failure of the patient to properly metabolise the amino acid phenylalanine owing to a deficiency of the enzyme phenylalanine hydroxylase necessary for its proper metabolism. Screening procedures for the detection of phenylketonuria in the neonatal period are available; these are the Guthrie bacterial inhibition assay test and a fluorimetric test. It is necessary for the infant to be on a normal milk diet prior to the test; therefore the test is usually done on the sixth or seventh day after birth using a small amount of blood obtained by heel prick. Confirmation of the disease is made by finding elevation of the phenylalanine level in the blood serum (normal level is 0·20 umol per litre of blood). Another screening method used before the introduction of the Guthrie test was the finding of phenylpyruvic acid in the urine using the Phenistix test or ferric chloride. Unfortunately this urine test may only become positive in these patients about four to six weeks after birth. If these patients are diagnosed sufficiently early the progress of the disease may be halted by the method of greatly reducing phenylalanine in the diet and thereby reducing the blood phenylalanine to normal levels. Various low-phenylalanine food preparations are available (Lofenalac, Minafen, Albumaid, Cymogran, Aminogran).

It is also necessary for pregnant women with elevated phenylalanine blood levels to have these high levels reduced to normal dietetically during pregnancy in order to protect the foetus from intrauterine damage.

Other inborn errors of metabolism may be detected early and dietetic control is possible in certain of these disorders. These include histidinaemia, tyrosinosis, homocystinuria and maple syrup urine disease. A dietetic preparation available for the control of histidinaemia is Cow and Gate Formula HF (2) and for tyrosinosis Cow and Gate Formula LPT (1) and LPTM (2).

14. Diseases of the Genitourinary System

In infancy and childhood this system may be affected by various disorders both congenital and acquired.

Disorders of the urine

Various abnormal constituents may be present in the urine. The presence of albumin may be shown by using a special test paper (Albustix); in the past its presence was detected by boiling or the salicylsulphonic acid test. Albumin occurs in patients with nephritis or nephrosis, in the presence of infection of the urinary tract, such as pyelitis, in cases of generalised infection with fever or as the condition of orthostatic or postural albuminuria. Orthostatic albuminuria is found in the older child occurring after much standing and is an innocuous condition; the early morning specimen of urine in these cases does not contain albumin. Blood in the urine (haematuria) may be caused by various conditions such as trauma to the kidney, acute nephritis, acute pyelocystitis, Wilm's tumour of the kidney, stone in the kidney, sulphonamide crystalluria, bilharzia of the bladder or by generalised blood diseases such as purpura or infections such as bacterial endocarditis. In some of these cases, the urine has a typical red or smoky appearance and shows red blood cells when examined microscopically. Red urine may also be due to haemoglobin (broken down red cells). In these cases there are no red cells in the urine; this condition may be due to congenital syphilis (paroxysmal haemoglobinuria), incompatible blood transfusions and other causes. Sugar (glucose) is present as an abnormal constituent of urine in cases of diabetes mellitus when acetone may also be found. The bile pigments such as bilirubin, urobilin and urobilinogen may be present in various types of jaundice.

Congenital abnormalities

The kidneys may be affected by different developmental abnormalities. They may be fused across the midline (horseshoe kidney) giving rise to obstruction to the ureters with the development of hydronephrosis. On rare occasions the kidneys may be absent or imperfectly formed (renal agenesis); if this condition is bilateral it is incompatible with survival and is often associated with a peculiar facial appearance described by Potter (Potter's facies) (Fig. 14.1). There is evidence to suggest that abnormality of formation or position of the

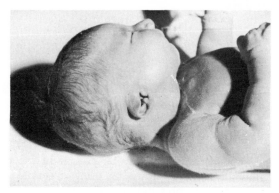

Fig. 14.1 Potter's facies. Note abnormal and low-placed ear; associated with renal agenesis.

external ears may be associated with abnormality of the renal system. Hydronephrosis (dilatation of the pelvis and kidney) may be present unilaterally or bilaterally (Fig. 14.2). It is due to some obstruction to the urinary tract such as congenital stricture, urethral valves or other abnormalities. The dilated part may be felt on abdominal palpation. The

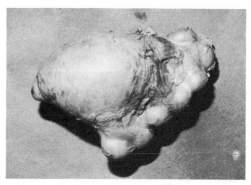

Fig. 14.2 Hydronephrosis of pelvis of ureter and kidney.

diagnosis should be confirmed by intravenous pyelography. The treatment requires relief of the obstruction if possible, otherwise removal of the affected part if unilateral. The ureters may also be abnormally dilated (hydroureter) due to some obstruction or other congenital abnormality such as a double ureter. The cases with obstruction are often associated with recurrent attacks of urinary infection and this infection will be cured only if the obstruction is surgically relieved. The very rare condition of congenital absence of the abdominal muscles ('prune belly' syndrome) is usually associated with severe abnormality and dilatation of the urinary system (Fig. 14.3). In patients with recurrent infections or other symptoms of urinary abnormality the possibility of the reflux of urine from the bladder up the ureter must be excluded by the use of a micturating cystogram.

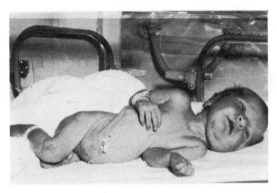

Fig. 14.3 'Prune belly' syndrome due to congenital absence of the abdominal muscles and often associated with severe congenital malformation of the urinary system.

Ectopia vesicae is a very rare congenital abnormality associated with absence of the anterior wall of the bladder and the lower abdominal wall (Fig. 14.4). These cases require elaborate surgery with transplantation of the ureters into the colon when the patient is a few years old or other surgical procedures.

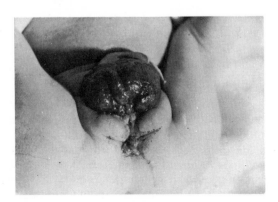

Fig. 14.4 Ectopia vesicae. An ectopic bladder.

Congenital polycystic disease of the kidneys is another rare congenital anomaly. These cases may be familial and may present clinically either in infancy or in adults over the age of about 40. The grossly enlarged kidneys may be felt in the loins and renal failure supervenes.

Pyelitis

This is an infection of the pelvis of the kidney and is frequently associated with involvement of the kidney itself (pyelonephritis) and the bladder (pyelocystitis). The condition may affect any age-group and recurrent attacks are often associated with some obstructive lesion of the urinary tract. The infection is most frequently due to the *Escherichia coli* organism. The onset may be acute in infancy with irritability, pyrexia (rigors) and diarrhoea. In the older child abdominal pain is often a feature. This pain starts in the loin and may pass to the inguinal region—frequency and burning on micturition being further clinical symptoms. The diagnosis may be confirmed by finding pus cells microscopically in a specimen of urine collected under sterile precautions. During the acute attack fluids should be given in quantity to these patients and the urine may be alkalinised with potassium citrate, but it is of paramount importance to use antimicrobial therapy such as the combination of trimethoprim and sulphamethoxazole or other sulphonamide drugs, nitrofurantoin (Furadantin), nalidixic acid or other suitable drug as indicated by bacteriological sensitivity tests. In recurrent attacks of pyelitis it is essential to exclude a congenital abnormality of the urinary tract by intravenous pyelography and a micturating cystogram. It is necessary to stress the need to exclude possible urinary infection by culturing the urine and having a bacteriological assessment of the viable count of infecting organism. Screening procedures are available to detect symptomless bacteriuria and these methods are being made available to certain susceptible groups of individuals such as pregnant women, schoolgirls and others (Uriglox, Uricult).

Acute nephritis

This is a common disease and often follows a Lancefield group A β-haemolytic streptococcal sore throat. It is often due to type 12 of this organism and occasionally 4, 25 or 49. The sore throat usually precedes the nephritis by about 10 to 14 days. The disease usually starts suddenly with haematuria (blood in the urine), giving a smoky appearance to the urine. Pyrexia may be present and the patient frequently has some puffiness of the face and swelling of the hands and feet. The blood pressure may be normal or raised and vomiting may occur. On rare occasions the patient develops drowsiness and convulsions with a high rise in the blood pressure (hypertensive encephalopathy). The urine is red and contains much albumin and blood and the amount passed is often diminished (oliguria). The blood urea is raised in some cases (normal blood urea 2·5 to 6·5 mmol per litre), the sedimentation rate is also increased and the antistreptolysin 0 titre (ASO) often elevated and the serum complement (C_3) lowered. These cases frequently recover completely (more than 85 per cent of cases). The acute disease may be complicated on rare occasions by hypertensive encephalopathy as mentioned above, by cardiac failure and by renal failure and anuria. In the few cases that do not recover completely the disease may linger slowly on towards the chronic stage of nephritis with hypertension, poor renal function and a raised blood urea.

There is no specific therapy for acute nephritis, but bed rest is necessary until the condition is quiescent. In the initial stages, the diet should be light with fluids only; when the haematuria has disappeared the diet may be increased with the gradual introduction of solids with protein. The throat infection should be treated with penicillin. The child should be kept at rest until evidence of activity has disappeared; this evidence includes the albuminuria, haematuria, oliguria, oedema, raised blood pressure, raised blood urea and raised sedimentation rate. The complication of hypertensive encephalopathy requires the use of sedation and the anti-hypertensive drugs, such as hydrallazine (Apresoline), guanethidine (Ismelin), methyldopa and others. Cardiac failure requires the usual therapeutic measures. In the management of chronic nephritis a controlled low-protein diet is necessary. The use of repeated haemodialysis (artificial kidney) is available as a method of treatment and further developments in the management of severe chronic nephritis are in the field of renal transplantation, which is meeting with success in children.

Nephrosis (Figs 14.5 and 14.6)

This is an uncommon disease with different causes. This condition is found at all ages and a rare severe congenital form has been recognised in Finland where it appears to be transmitted as an autosomal recessive hereditary disease. The disease is made up clinically of four main features:

1. Oedema
2. Albuminuria
3. Hypoalbuminaemia
4. Hypercholesterolaemia

The oedema is of gradual onset and is usually the first thing which brings the child to the doctor. It is present in the face, with puffiness below the eyes, at the ankles, and in the peritoneal cavity, producing ascites. This oedema is probably caused by the lowered osmotic pressure of the blood due to the low serum albumin, and also by salt retention.

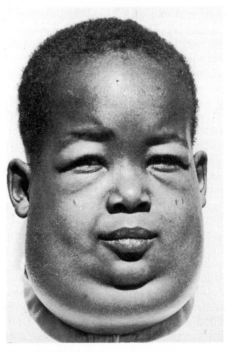

Fig. 14.5 Gross oedema in nephrosis.

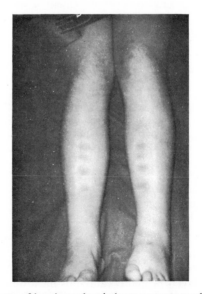

Fig. 14.6 Pitting oedema of legs in nephrosis (note pressure marks of fingers).

The patient passes from 5 to 20 g of albumin in the urine daily, which may be estimated by using an Esbach's albuminometer. The blood serum which contains protein in the form of albumin and globulins is affected by a reduction in the serum albumin and a rise in the a_2-globulin. The lipoid metabolism of the patient is affected and this is shown by the high blood cholesterol level (sometimes up to 26 mmol per litre). The disease is of insidious onset and is very protracted. Some of these children may recover completely or they may develop signs of renal failure with hypertension and high blood urea levels.

Treatment

Treatment is related to the following basic principles:

1. Maintaining adequate nutrition, by offering the patient a high protein low-sodium (up to 3 g of protein per kg bodyweight per day).

2. Eliminating oedema. There is no specific method for this, but various measures have been adopted to produce a diuresis in these patients. The corticosteroids such as the cortisone derivatives (e.g. prednisone, prednisolone) or ACTH should be used in the treatment of nephrosis and with this corticosteroid therapy the prognosis has much improved and many patients with this syndrome are being cured. The ascites should be tapped only if it interferes mechanically with the patient's well being. It is remarkable that an attack of measles may produce a remission in these patients. In the patients who do not respond to corticosteroid therapy the use of the immunosuppressive drugs such as cyclophosphamide often has success.

3. Prevention of infection. These cases have a great tendency to develop pneumococcal infections, especially peritonitis, which may have a fatal termination. Fortunately these infections may be adequately prevented and treated with penicillin and other antibiotics.

Acute renal failure

In this condition the urinary output is greatly reduced (oliguria) and often becomes completely suppressed (anuria). It may follow sulphonamide crystalluria (blockage by sulphonamide crystals in the urine) or necrosis of the renal tubules associated with incompatible blood transfusion, crush injuries, burns or shock. The blood urea and serum potassium levels rise and these patients become listless, drowsy and comatose. It is recognised that the kidney disease process is reversible providing that these patients can be kept alive. The treatment requires the prevention of overhydration by carefully controlling the fluid intake to replace only the 'invisible' fluid loss via the skin and respiratory system plus any urinary output volume and stool fluid loss. Sufficient calories must be given but no protein. Peritoneal dialysis is a necessary and effective form of treatment, and disposable aids for this therapy are available; haemodialysis is seldom needed.

Haemolytic-uraemic syndrome (Gasser's syndrome)

This condition is an extremely serious disease affecting infants. These patients usually present with a diarrhoea and develop marked pallor (due to an acute haemolytic process) and also uraemia (due to renal failure). They have thrombocytopenia (reduced platelets) and become extremely ill. The red blood cells have a typical fragmented appearance. There is a high mortality with this disease. Symptomatic management is necessary and this may require dialysis and blood transfusion. On the basis of this condition being possibly related to a process of intravascular coagulation, heparin is also used in the treatment of this disease with varying results. Corticosteroid therapy has also been used without much benefit.

Tumours (Fig. 14.7)

Wilm's tumour (nephroblastoma) is the commonest renal tumour of childhood. It occurs in young children and may present clinically as an abdominal swelling. On abdominal palpation, the tumour is felt in the loin; haematuria may occur. This tumour is very malignant and may spread to the lungs and other parts of the body with a fatal termination.

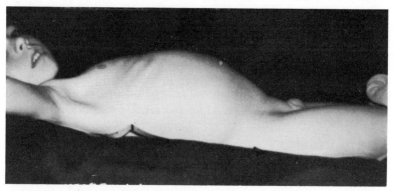

Fig. 14.7 Photograph of child showing distension of the abdomen due to the presence of a Wilms' tumour (nephroblastoma).

Intravenous pyelography shows abnormality of the pelvis of the kidney and X-ray examination of the chest may indicate the spread of the tumour to the lungs. These cases require urgent treatment in the form of surgical removal of the affected kidney followed by radiation therapy and chemotherapy. This form of treatment may be successful in some cases although the prognosis is poor. Improved results are being obtained where surgery is combined with radiation therapy and chemotherapy and the drugs that are used include actinomycin D (Cosmegen Lyovac) and vincristine (Oncovin).

Vulvovaginitis

This condition may be caused by the *Gonococcus, Streptococcus* or *Pneumococcus*, or it may be associated with threadworm infestation. The main symptom is a vaginal discharge with painful micturition. A swab is essential to detect the causative organism, and treatment requires cleanliness of the affected parts in addition to the use of chemo- and antibiotic therapy.

Undescended testicle

This condition must be differentiated from a retracted testicle which may be replaced easily in the scrotal sac. Various types of this condition occur, such as the testicle retained in the abdominal cavity, the type in an ectopic abnormal site and the type with the testicle in the inguinal canal. The last-mentioned variety is the commonest. Hormone therapy is not successful in treating this problem; surgical replacement (orchidopexy) is the best form of treatment.

Phimosis

In this rare condition the prepuce is tight and cannot be retracted over the glans penis. If it is sufficiently severe to obstruct the urinary flow circumcision is necessary. This operation is also done for religious

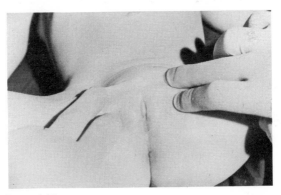

Fig. 14.8 Adherent labia.

reasons. On rare occasions the prepuce is retracted and cannot be replaced (paraphimosis) with the production of a swollen inflamed glans. This requires urgent treatment to reduce the swelling—local applications may succeed but surgical intervention may be necessary to reduce the paraphimosis.

Bilharzia (schistosomiasis)

The parasite *Schistosoma haematobium* produces eggs with a terminal spike. This worm infests the urinary tract and the eggs are excreted in the urine and produce lesions of the ureters and bladder with the typical symptom of terminal haematuria (blood in the urine at the end of micturition). The schistosoma in its life-cycle requires to pass through a snail and then enter man as an embryo cercaria to produce the disease. The early invasive phase may produce a transient fever (Katayama fever) and later the disease develops. It occurs extensively in different parts of the world, such as South and Central Africa, and Egypt, and snail-infested waters in endemic areas are dangerous to man. Another type of schistosoma (*Schistosoma mansoni*) may also infest man and usually affects the bowel producing rectal bleeding as a symptom. Treatment is difficult, but intravenous antimony may meet with great success; apart from sodium antimony tartrate, sodium antimonylgluconate (Triostam) is also useful as an intravenous drug. A schistosomicide preparation useful in the treatment of this disease is niridazole (Ambilhar) administered orally. Another orally administered drug for the treatment of this disease is lucanthone (Miracil D) but antimony is the most effective drug available.

15. Diseases of the Nervous System

The central nervous system may be affected by many different diseases. The brain and spinal cord are covered by three membranes or meninges, from within outwards (a) the pia mater, (b) the arachnoid and (c) the outer covering of the dura mater. The pia mater is a vascular membrane lying in contact with the brain. The arachnoid is a thin avascular membrane, and external to it lies the dura mater, a thick membrane which, with its septa of the falx cerebri and tentorium cerebelli, supports the whole brain mass. The cerebrospinal fluid circulates around the brain and spinal cord in the space between the pia and arachnoid (subarachnoid space) and has its origin from the choroid plexus in the lateral ventricles of the brain. Cerebrospinal fluid may be obtained for examination by the procedure of lumbar puncture, when a needle is inserted into the subarachnoid space in the lumbar region, usually between the third and fourth lumbar vertebrae or one space lower. Normally the cerebrospinal fluid is clear and colourless and does not coagulate; it has fewer than five lymphocytes per mm³. The protein content is normally between 0·15–0·45 g/l and the sugar content 2·24–3·36 mmol/l.

Meningitis (Fig. 15.1)

This inflammatory condition of the meninges is not uncommon; it usually affects the pia and arachnoid and is known as a leptomeningitis. Various bacteria may produce the disease, the commonest types in childhood being the meningococcus, pneumococcus, *Haemophilus influenzae* and the tubercle bacillus. Less common types are the streptococcal and staphycoccal varieties. In the newborn age-group a coliform meningitis is probably the commonest type. Congenital syphilis may also rarely produce a meningitis in the young infant.

Tuberculous meningitis has been discussed in another section.

Meningococcal meningitis (cerebrospinal fever)

This condition may occur sporadically or in epidemic form. It is due to a Gram-negative diplococcus, the meningococcus (*Neisseria meningitidis*), and has its origin in the nasopharynx from whence it invades the bloodstream and may produce a petechial skin eruption (spotted fever). The infection settles in the meninges producing an acute inflammatory reaction, with the formation of cloudy, turbid cerebrospinal fluid; this may be obtained for diagnostic purposes by lumbar puncture. (The fluid has a raised protein and lowered sugar content, many pus cells and the meningococcus organism may be obtained by suitable smears and by culture.) The child is acutely ill, pyrexial, has a headache, often vomits, may have convulsions and shows signs of meningeal irritation such as

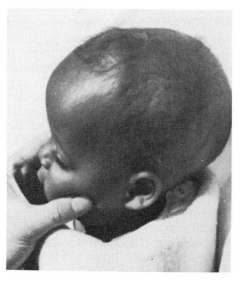

Fig. 15.1 Tense prominent anterior fontanelle due to increased intracranial pressure.

neck rigidity and head retraction, and a positive Kernig's sign (pain and stiffness in the hamstring muscles on attempting to extend the leg at the knee joint with the hip flexed). The organism may be obtained by blood culture, but the diagnosis is confirmed by lumbar puncture and obtaining cerebrospinal fluid for examination.

This disease requires careful nursing and adequate care for the nutrition of the patient. The sulphonamide drugs such as sulphadiazine were specific for this infection although resistant strains do occur. Penicillin is also effective and is the drug of choice. Sulphadiazine must be given in adequate dosage, orally if possible but by parenteral means if oral therapy is impossible due to excessive vomiting. Penicillin must be used in suitable dosage for the treatment of this infection. Various complications such as deafness or arthritis may occur. Close contacts of a case of meningococcal meningitis can be protected from contracting the disease by administering a short course of rifampicin, sulpha drug or penicillin.

An extremely severe form of septicaemia may occur with a meningococcal infection known as the Friderichsen-Waterhouse syndrome. It is a fulminating condition with a high mortality. It has an acute onset with an extensive purpuric eruption covering almost the whole body, and extreme shock with a low blood pressure. This septicaemia is associated with suprarenal haemorrhages and urgent therapy is essential if an attempt is to be made to save these patients. Intravenous fluids, massive antibiotic and chemotherapy are necessary and corticosteroids may be helpful. Heparin may also be useful if an intravascular coagulation defect occurs.

Influenzal meningitis

This type of meningitis, due to the organism *Haemophilus influenzae* (type B), affects infants usually under the age of 2 years. It is an extremely serious form of meningeal infection, and was always fatal before the present therapeutic drugs were available. The illness usually starts acutely, with vomiting, irritability, pyrexia and convulsions. Lumbar puncture confirms the diagnosis as the cerebrospinal fluid is turbid and has many pus cells with a raised protein and reduced sugar content; the *Haemophilus* may be found on direct smear or on culture.

This disease requires urgent treatment with the use of ampicillin and other antibiotics such as streptomycin, the tetracyclines or cephaloridine or a sulpha drug. Chloramphenicol is highly effective in the treatment of this disease but because of its side-effects should be reserved for cases which are resistant to the other available agents. Sensitivity tests are done on the organism to assess the best combination of antimicrobial agents to use in the effective control of this serious infection. If much vomiting is present intravenous fluid therapy is necessary. In some cases of this type of meningitis (and other forms of pyogenic meningitis) a subdural collection of fluid may occur as a complication. This effusion of fluid in the subdural space surrounding the brain must be removed by needling, and later possibly by some neurosurgical procedure.

Pneumococcal meningitis

This type of infection of the meninges is due to the pneumococcus (Gram-positive diplococci) and may spread from other pneumococcal infections in the body such as an otitis media. It is a very serious disease and was formerly always fatal. Signs of meningeal irritation are present and lumbar puncture confirms the diagnosis. This infection produces the typical greenish-yellow pus associated with pneumococcal infections.

The drugs of choice in this disease are sulphadiazine in maximum dosage together with very high dosage, frequently administered, intramuscular penicillin therapy (e.g. one million units of crystalline penicillin G two-hourly by the intravenous or intramuscular route).

This form of therapy has superseded the necessity of giving penicillin intrathecally into the subarachnoid space in the lumbar region (2500 to 10,000 units of crystalline penicillin G well diluted).

Other less common forms of meningitis such as those due to the streptococcus, staphylococcus or the *Escherichia coli* in the newborn period require the appropriate chemotherapeutic or antibiotic agents. All cases of meningitis of necessity require expert nursing care if success in treatment is to be obtained.

Encephalitis

This disease has become more common and may be caused by a virus infection, such as that of mumps, the coxsackie viruses or other known and unknown viruses. The patient has a headache, pyrexia and often shows signs of meningeal irritation. Lumbar puncture and examination of cerebrospinal fluid shows an increase in the cell count, usually lymphocytes, and an increase in the protein and a normal or raised sugar content.

There is no specific therapy for these diseases except careful and expert nursing and bed rest. A specific type of encephalitis may rarely complicate vaccination (commoner in a primary vaccination in an older child or an adolescent) or some of the acute infectious fevers such as measles and chickenpox. These conditions usually occur about 10 to 14 days after the primary condition, with the patient developing signs of meningeal irritation, such as neck rigidity, pyrexia, headache, vomiting and often convulsions. Some cases recover completely, but there is the danger of permanent sequelae, such as hemiplegias, occurring in a proportion of surviving cases. In this type of encephalitis the therapeutic use of human immunoglobulin and corticosteroid therapy may be helpful.

Poliomyelitis

This disease is caused by a virus infection affecting the anterior horn cells of the spinal cord. The virus is present in the stools and serious epidemics of the disease have occurred in most countries of the world. The infecting agent probably enters the bloodstream via the naso-pharynx and the bowel. Soon after tonsillectomy, patients may, if exposed to the disease, develop a severe form of bulbar paralysis; in view of this danger tonsillectomy should not be performed in the presence of an epidemic of poliomyelitis but with universal active immunisation this danger has been virtually removed.

The clinical features of the condition take on various forms but the commonest type of onset is with the child developing a coryzal condition with a mild pyrexia, sore throat and vomiting, followed by signs of neck and back stiffness with headache and apprehension. This may be followed by paralysis of any part of the body associated on occasion with spasm of muscles. The blood may show an increase in the white cells (leucocytosis). The examination of the cerebrospinal fluid in the early stages of the infection shows an increase in the cells, particularly lymphocytes; in the later stages of the disease the cell count tends to fall and the protein content rises. On rare occasions a patient, previously well, may wake in the morning with a paralysed limb.

Some cases of this disease do not develop paralysis and these may be called the abortive type. Immunity is conferred by the infection. There is no specific therapy for this infection, but much may be achieved by careful nursing and maintaining any paralysed part in a position of rest. Heat is useful in treating and relieving spasm. Intermittent positive pressure ventilators may be life-saving in cases with respiratory paralysis. In the later stages of the condition, where the acute phase has subsided, physiotherapy is essential in the treatment of paralysed muscles. Paralysed parts, with expert treatment, may show improvement for about two years. Later, orthopaedic management is necessary in achieving maximum function of paralysed limbs. As mentioned elsewhere in this book, an immunising poliomyelitis vaccine for general use is available; the Salk vaccine (a killed virus vaccine) was available for administration by intramuscular injection but this has been almost universally replaced by the Sabin-type (an attenuated live virus vaccine containing the three polioviruses types I, II and III) which is administered by the oral route for active immunisation. In the past human immunoglobulin has been used to produce passive immunisation of susceptible contacts in the presence of an epidemic of poliomyelitis.

Much stress was laid on the occurrence of paralysis in a limb in which injections such as alum-containing immunisation preparations have been given; with the extensive poliomyelitis immunisation being undertaken this is no longer a problem.

Cerebral tumour

These tumours may occur in childhood; the majority are situated below the tentorium cerebelli (subtentorial) in the cerebellum but they also occur in other situations. They may be benign or malignant. The medulloblastoma of the cerebellum is the commonest malignant type. Headache and vomiting are common symptoms. These tumours produce evidence of increased intracranial pressure such as papilloedema and widening of the sutures. The EMI brain scanner is used to undertake computerised axial tomography using a low radiation dosage equivalent to a lateral skull radiograph. This procedure is extremely useful to detect intracranial tumours, subdural effusions, hydrocephalus and other diseases. Neurosurgical treatment is essential in the management of these patients.

Cerebral palsy

This condition has received much attention and great advances have been made in the management of these affected children. There are various types of cerebral palsy such as the spastic paralysis (cerebral diplegia) with or without abnormal movements of an athetoid or choreiform nature, the atonic type or the hemiplegic type. These cases may be due to prenatal causes such as congenital abnormality of the brain, natal causes such as the asphyxial and anoxic states of birth, kernicterus or cerebral haemorrhage, or postnatal causes such as trauma or encephalitis. It is important to realise that many cases of cerebral palsy have normal intelligence and normal mental development, and this fact makes it important that all facilities be available for their proper care and training. This management requires a team effort with the co-operation of the parents, the paediatrician, the family doctor, the orthopaedic surgeon, social worker, nurse, physiotherapist, speech therapist, psychologist and educationalist.

Hydrocephalus (Figs 15.2, 15.3 and 15.4)

In order to appreciate this condition it is necessary to have knowledge of the formation and circulation of cerebrospinal fluid. This fluid is formed by the choroid plexus in the lateral ventricles; it then circulates from these ventricles via the foramina of Monro to the centrally placed third ventricle; from this point the cerebrospinal fluid passes through the aqueduct of Silvius to the fourth ventricle and from this space it passes through the lateral and medial foramina (foramina of Luschka and Magendie) into the cisterna magna at the base of the brain and the subarachnoid space over the brain and spinal cord. It is then absorbed by the arachnoid granulations on the superior surface of the brain. Hydrocephalus is associated with abnormal amounts of cerebrospinal fluid in the brain and enlargement of the ventricular system. This condition is usually due to some obstruction to the flow of cerebrospinal fluid or to interference with its absorption and may give rise to much enlargement of the head. The pressure and enlargement of the ventricles causes thinning and destruction of brain tissue. The causes of the obstructive lesion may be a congenital abnormality of the ventricular system (e.g. congenital obstruction of the aqueduct of Silvius), a birth injury with cerebral haemorrhage, intrauterine infection with the protozoa *Toxoplasma gondii* (congenital toxoplasmosis) or a postnatal acquired disease such as meningitis or a tumour. Various operative procedures have been attempted in the treatment of this condition; an operation of anastomosing the subarachnoid space to a ureter (arachno-ureterostomy) or the peritoneal cavity has been done; polythene tubing has been used for this anastomosis which allows for the drainage of cerebrospinal fluid. The most favoured operation with good results is a

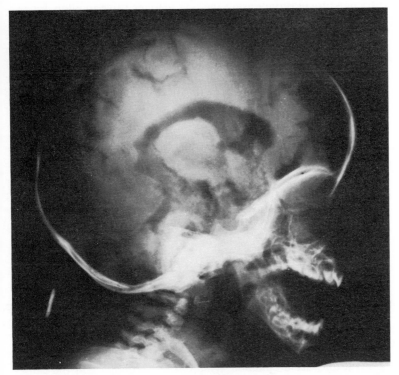

Fig. 15.2 Lateral X-ray of skull with an air encephalogram showing dilatation of the ventricular system and atrophy of the brain.

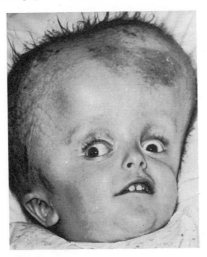

Fig. 15.3 Extreme form of hydrocephalus; note the eyes pushed down.

ventriculo-auriculostomy using the Spitz-Holter valve to allow for the proper flow of cerebrospinal fluid along the cannulas used to connect the lateral ventricle to the jugular vein and the right auricle of the heart.

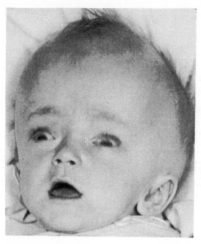

Fig. 15.4 Another case of hydrocephalus.

Convulsions and epilepsy

Convulsions are a common symptom in childhood and the causes may be of different origin. It has been said that about 5 per cent of all children have convulsions before the age of 5 years; a large proportion of these occur in the infant over 6 months of age. Convulsions may be divided into those due to a definite organic cause, those associated with pyrexia and those due to idiopathic epilepsy. It must be stressed that convulsions are a symptom. The organic causes of convulsions may be those that follow cerebral trauma whether from birth or in later years, congenital abnormality of the brain, infections of the central nervous system such as meningitis and encephalitis, low blood calcium (rickets) and cerebral tumours. Other organic causes may be associated with hypoglycaemia and attention has also been directed to possible pyridoxine (vitamin B_6) deficiency as a cause of infantile convulsions. In the infant over the age of 6 months, many cases of convulsions are associated with a fever usually over $38.9°C$ ($102°F$). This pyrexia may be due to any cause and the convulsions are usually of the major variety. Idiopathic epilepsy may manifest itself in different ways:

1. Grand mal or major seizures
2. Petit mal or minor seizures
3. Jacksonian seizures which are focal in nature affecting only a part of the patient, such as an arm or leg

4. Psychomotor epilepsy, where the patient has attacks of abnormal behaviour

Grand mal attacks are always associated with the typical fit. These attacks have a tonic phase with spasm of muscles followed by the clonic phase with its sharp jerky movements when the patient may pass urine

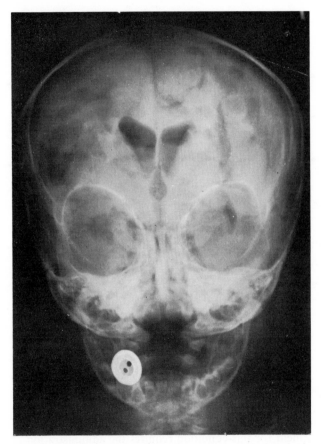

Fig. 15.5 Air encephalogram showing the outline of the lateral and third ventricles and also air in the subarachnoid space over the brain surface.

and bite his tongue. This is followed by a period of unconsciousness which passes into sleep. On rare occasions these major seizures continue as a status epilepticus, which may be dangerous to the patient if not relieved. Petit mal attacks are associated with a momentary loss of consciousness lasting up to 30 seconds. The patient usually stops his activities during the attack and then resumes what he was doing previously. The attacks may be extremely frequent, up to about 20 or more a day. These cases of epilepsy may be confirmed by electro-encephalographic tracings (Figs 15.6 and 15.7). Infantile spasm is a condition seen in infancy which may be associated with myoclonic seizures and the so-called 'salaam' attacks. This condition has an extremely

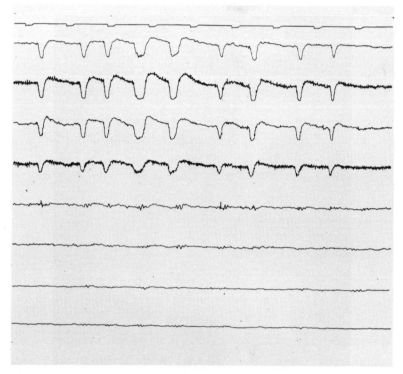

Fig. 15.6 A normal eight-channel electroencephalographic tracing recorded with the eyes open.

disorganised EEG pattern known as hypsarrythmia which is diagnostic. The treatment for this condition requires the administration of ACTH or other corticosteroid preparation. This treatment often improves the attacks but unfortunately in many cases mental subnormality ensues.

The treatment of epilepsy or convulsions in general requires the control of the seizure; for this purpose various drugs are available. The usual drugs used in the control of major attacks are phenobarbitone and soluble phenytoin (Epanutin, Dilantin), other useful drugs in epilepsy are primidone (Mysoline), sulthiame (Ospolot) and carbamaze-pine (Tegretol). For petit mal attacks the drug ethosuximide (Zarontin) is effective in most cases; other useful drugs for the treatment of petit

mal attacks are acetazolamide (Diamox), troxidone (Tridione) and
paramethadione (Paradione). For an attack of status epilepticus it is
essential that the seizures be brought under control as quickly as possible
and for this purpose diazepam (Valium) or paraldehyde are useful. In
very severe cases where the attack becomes uncontrollable it may be
necessary to use general anaesthesia.

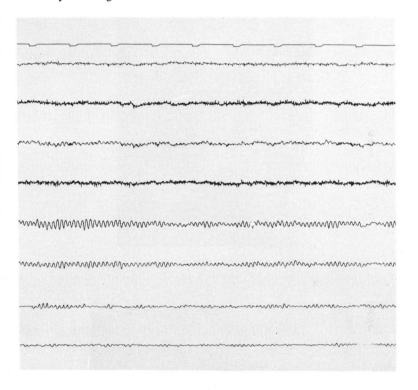

Fig. 15.7 A normal eight-channel electroencephalographic tracing recorded with the
eyes closed.

Spina bifida

This is a congenital abnormality associated with absence of closure
of certain parts of the vertebral canal. There are various types such as
spina bifida occulta, which is the commonest variety and has only a
defect in the vertebral bone, usually situated in the lumbar region and
may only be detected by X-ray examination; meningocele, a defect
associated with a swelling containing cerebrospinal fluid usually
situated in the lumbar region and less commonly in the cervical area. If
the sac contains the spinal cord and nerve fibres, the lesion is called a

meningomyelocele (Fig. 15.8). A more severe condition is a myelocele where the central canal is open at the body surface (Fig. 15.9). These extreme cases may be associated with paralysis of the lower limbs, of the anal sphincter and of bladder control. The management of these cases, except spina bifida occulta which does not require treatment, is

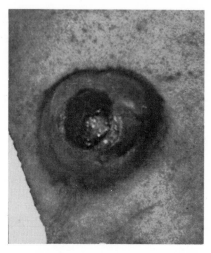

Fig. 15.8 A meningomyelocele in the lumbar region.

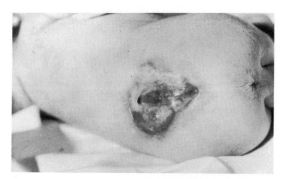

Fig. 15.9 Lumbar meningomyelocele in a newborn male infant.

surgical and operation should be done only in selected cases as early as possible; unfortunately, following surgical repair of cases of meningocele, these patients often develop hydrocephalus. This complication, however, may now be better controlled with the operation of a ventriculoauriculostomy using the Spitz-Holter valve.

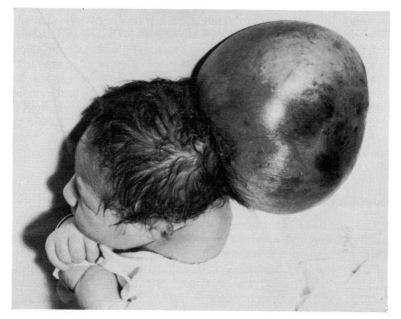

Fig. 15.10 An encephalocele.

Polyneuritis

All forms of polyneuritis are uncommon in childhood. The condition may be caused by diphtheria, heavy metal poisoning (e.g. arsenic) and virus infections. Acute infective polyneuritis (Guillain-Barré syndrome) is a disease probably caused by a virus infection; this condition is associated with evidence of polyneuritis affecting different nerves producing such signs as a facial palsy and peripheral paralyses. The cerebrospinal fluid in these cases has a markedly raised protein content but a normal cell count. The outlook is usually good in that they eventually recover after many months. Diphtheric polyneuritis may complicate cases of diphtheria and usually produces three types of paralyses. These paralyses affect the soft palate, with regurgitation of food through the nose and a nasal voice, the eye muscles of accommodation and the peripheral paralyses often affecting the leg muscles.

Pink disease (acrodynia)

This disease, now uncommon, affects infants from about 6 to 24 months. The cause is probably mercury poisoning (some teething powders in the past have contained mercury in the form of calomel). Other possible aetiological factors previously considered were a virus infection or some deficiency state. The clinical picture is one of an extremely irritable child with cold, pink, swollen hands and feet and excessive sweating producing a typical sweat rash. Other manifestations include photophobia with the child burrowing his head into the pillow to avoid the light, tachycardia, raised blood pressure (hypertension), stomatitis, hypotonia and extreme anorexia. These infants are the despair of their parents as the disease is so prolonged (up to 6 months) before recovery takes place. If possible they should not be admitted to hospital due to the danger of cross-infection. Various therapeutic measures have been adopted; these include dimercaprol in cases associated with mercury poisoning, belladonna and sedation in addition to careful nursing.

Bornholm disease (epidemic pleurodynia)

This condition is an acute muscle disease (myalgia) which affects mainly the diaphragm, producing severe pain especially with breathing. There is pyrexia and frequently abdominal pain. The disease is due to infection with the Coxsackie B virus and may occur in epidemic form. The prognosis is good and treatment requires bed rest and good nursing; there is no specific therapy available.

Tetanus

This is a serious disease due to an anaerobic spore-forming organism, *Clostridium tetani*. The disease follows wound contamination by this organism and the infection remains localised; the severe systemic features of the disease are due to a powerful exotoxin liberated by the organism. The incubation period is from 5 to 14 days, but may be prolonged, and the onset is insidious with increasing muscle stiffness developing. This affects mainly the jaw and neck and is followed by difficulty in opening the mouth (trismus). There is difficulty in swallowing and clonic convulsions (which may be initiated by the slightest stimulus) occur. These muscles develop spasm and there may be board-like rigidity of the abdomen; the facial muscles also take part in this generalised spasm with the development of the typical 'risus sardonicus' (sardonic smile). The mortality is high. Active immunisation with tetanus toxoid is essential in preventing this serious disease and is an absolutely necessary preventive medical procedure. In the unimmunised wounded individual passive immunisation with human tetanus immunoglobulin (Humotet) is necessary to prevent the development of this disease. In the past before human tetanus immunoglobulin was available it was the practice to use tetanus antitoxin (ATS) which could cause severe reactions in patients sensitive to horse serum. The usual dose of human tetanus immunoglobulin for passive immunisation is 250 i.u. but this could be increased to 500 i.u. if there is a risk of heavy contamination with *Clostridium tetani* or if a period longer than 24 hours has elapsed since the wound was sustained. In the management of a patient with tetanus, sedation, muscle relaxants, penicillin and human tetanus immunoglobulin are necessary in addition to expert intensive nursing care. It may also be necessary to use tracheostomy and a ventilator in addition to the other procedures. The dosage of human tetanus immunoglobulin for the treatment of tetanus is 30 to 300 i.u. per kg bodyweight given intramuscularly.

Myasthenia gravis

In this condition there is weakness of muscles. Excessive fatigue follows continual muscle contractions and this fatigue improves on rest. It may occur as a specific disease and may also be associated with other conditions such as hyperthyroidism and muscular dystrophy. The cause is unknown although there may be an association with enlargement of the thymus gland. It appears to be due to interference with neuromuscular transmission of impulses or a block at the end-plate; it responds to anticholinesterase drugs. It is rare in childhood and is commoner in females. It may have its onset in late childhood. The commonest sign is ptosis (drooping of the eyelids) and ophthalmoplegias (paralysis or weakness of the eye muscles) may occur. There may also be difficulty in swallowing, a nasal voice and weakness of the arms and legs. These symptoms improve on rest or following sleep and worsen with increased activity and also with infections. A diagnostic test is the response to the intravenous injection of edrophonium (Tensilon) in a dosage of 5 to 10 mg; this is followed by a rapid brief improvement in the symptoms. Treatment is based on the response to neostigmine (Prostigmin) or its related drug pyridostigmine (Mestinon) or distigmine (Ubretid) and these are administered by mouth to maintain improvement. If a thymic tumour (thymoma) is present it should be removed. A temporary neonatal form of myasthenia gravis may occur in the newborn child born to a mother who has this disease.

Migraine

This condition is seen in childhood and has similar symptoms to the condition in adults with the paroxysmal headache usually one-sided, nausea and visual symptoms. There is often a family history of this condition and the attacks in childhood are often of shorter duration; abdominal pain may also be seen in childhood. Similar measures to those taken in the adult are adopted for these attacks.

There are other extremely rare neurological and muscle diseases such as the familial hereditary ataxias, e.g. Friedreich's ataxia, progressive spinal muscular atrophy (Werdnig-Hoffman disease), pseudomyopathic spinal muscular atrophy (Kugelberg-Welander syndrome), benign

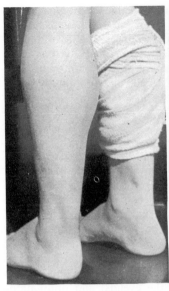
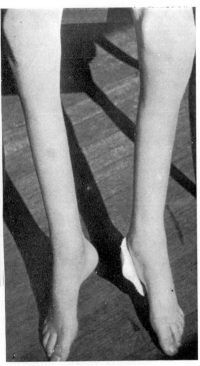

Fig. 15.11 Large calves of a patient with pseudohypertrophic muscular dystrophy of the Duchenne type (wasted muscle replaced by fat).

Fig. 15.12 Marked symmetrical wasting of the muscles of the leg due to the rare disease of peroneal muscular atrophy (Marie-Charcot-Tooth type).

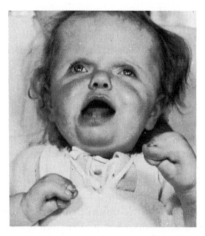

Fig. 15.13 Rare condition of acrocephalosyndactyly showing the gross abnormality of the hands with fused fingers, and the skull abnormality of oxycephaly ('tower skull').

congenital hypotonia ('floppy baby'), the myopathies (pseudohyper-trophic muscular dystrophy, Duchenne type) and others but these are rare and will not be considered further.

Various uncommon abnormalities of the skull are described. Oxy-cephaly ('tower skull') (Fig. 15.13) is one type where the skull is dome-shaped; other types include the long narrow skull (scaphocephaly) and the asymmetrical type (plagiocephaly). Some of these abnormalities are due to abnormal and early fusion of certain sutures of the skull (cranio-synostosis, craniostenosis) and may be associated with increased intracranial pressure which may require neurosurgical relief. The rare facial abnormalities such as craniofacial dysostosis (Crouzon's disease) and ocular hypertelorism are being surgically corrected by extensive operative procedures devised by Tessier.

Subacute sclerosing (or inclusion) panencephalitis

This is a very rare fatal neurological disorder. The symptoms include slow mental deterioration associated with paralysis and extrapyramidal signs with myoclonic or athetoid movements of the limbs. The particular interest of this condition is the finding of the measles virus in the brain tissue and also that these patients develop very high measles antibody levels in the blood and cerebrospinal fluid; there is often a history of these patients having had an attack of measles a long time previous to this fatal neurological disease developing.

Wilson's disease (hepatolenticular degeneration)

This disease is a rare inborn error of copper metabolism and is a hereditary condition transmitted as an autosomal recessive (where the risk of a similar disease affecting a sibling of a patient is one in four). An excess of copper accumulates in various tissues including the brain, liver, kidney and cornea and the defect involves a reduction of the main copper-containing plasma protein, caeruloplasmin (an α_2-globulin). In the clinical pattern of Wilson's disease there is evidence of liver disease in certain cases and neurological involvement where speech may be affected and become slurred; there is also drooling of saliva and the patient often has a rather fixed stare, increased tone and rigidity of the limbs and mental deterioration (Fig. 15.14). A very important clinical sign is the development of brown discoloration of the cornea (in Descemet's membrane of the cornea) due to the deposition of copper; this sign is known as the Kayser-Fleischer ring and can usually be detected by the use of a slit lamp. The treatment of this condition requires control of the copper intake and decreasing the total body-store of copper. Potassium sulphide assists in reducing bowel absorption of copper; in addition chelating agents assist in the excretion of body copper. These agents include D-penicillamine (Distamine, Cuprimine) which is administered by mouth and is extremely useful in improving the clinical pattern of this disease. Other chelating agents such as dimercaprol may also be used, administered by intramuscular injection.

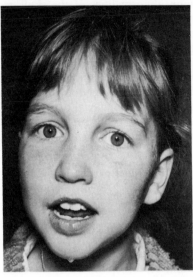

Fig. 15.14 Wilson's disease illustrating the fixed facial expression with dribbling of saliva.

Cerebral gigantism

This is a rare syndrome described by Sotos in 1962. These patients are large at birth, being usually above the ninetieth centile for length and weight and have a high rate of growth which continues and is followed by an early puberty with an increased rate of dental development. They have a characteristic appearance of head and face with the head being large and the length of the head being greater than the breadth. There is prominence of the forehead with deep-set eyes, high-arched palate, large ears and jaw and a tendency to having clumsy movements. The cause is not known and there is a possibility of abnormal cerebral regulation of growth.

16. Functional Nervous Disorders

There are numerous nervous disorders functional in origin which affect children. The proper psychological upbringing and control of any growing infant and child is essential for their proper care. A child requires security as the basis for his normal development and this security is found under normal circumstances in the environmental surroundings of the home and family. The father, mother and child may be graphically described as forming a triangle with a link between the three. If these links are broken or upset for any reason, the effect on the child may produce any functional nervous disorder; this break in any part of the triangle immediately upsets the feeling of security which every child requires. Examples of these upsets in the links of this triangle may be any cause of a broken home such as divorce or the arrival of another child in the family. Various common disorders of this nature will now be briefly discussed.

Thumb-sucking

This habit is extremely common and is usually most marked in the tired infant before sleep. The condition does not do much harm and it is even doubtful whether it plays any part in the production of protruding teeth. The thumb itself may develop thickened skin and callosities. It usually disappears in the second year but may persist much longer.

Disorders of sleep

Disturbed sleep occurs frequently in infants and older children. In infancy it may be caused by hunger due to underfeeding, by painful eruption of teeth or any illness associated with pain or irritability. In the older child improper habits may give rise to difficulty in getting the child to sleep. The procedure of getting a child to sleep should be a routine happening and every effort must be made to avoid overexcitement or overeating before bedtime. Fear may cause sleeplessness in the child and this fear may be engendered by the foolish behaviour of the parents.

Night-terrors and nightmares may affect the older child; the affected person may wake up in the middle of the night with a screaming attack which is completely forgotten by morning.

Talking during sleep may occur in nervous children who may be under some strain such as competitive examinations.

Enuresis (bed-wetting)

This is an extremely common complaint and very difficult to manage. The wetting may occur only at night as nocturnal enuresis or also by day—the diurnal type. A minority of these cases are due to an organic condition such as diseases with polyuria (diabetes mellitus, diabetes insipidus and chronic nephritis), urinary tract infections or mental subnormality. Spina bifida occulta has been blamed as a cause for enuresis, but this congenital abnormality is not an aetiological factor. The greater number of cases of enuresis have a psychological background as the basis for this unfortunate and distressing condition. Some of these children have never had bladder control whereas others have developed control and later (at about 4 years of age) started wetting the bed.

In the management of this condition it is essential to exclude any organic basis for the disease; if such a cause is found it must be treated. The majority of cases with their psychological causes for the condition require careful handling on this basis. An attempt must be made to elucidate and treat any possible psychological factors and this requires sympathetic handling of the patient. There is no place for the harsh management of these children; every effort must be made to encourage the child and relieve any tension in the home environment. Simple measures such as withholding fluids from late afternoon and waking the child at different times of the night to empty his bladder may be useful. These children tend to be deep sleepers. Certain drugs such as amitriptyline (Tryptizol) or imipramine (Tofranil) may be useful in controlling this condition. In the past other drugs such as ephedrine and belladonna have been used. An alarm buzzer which wakens the child when wet may also be very useful in the management.

Head-banging

This condition affects infants and may be associated with mental subnormality or with some irritation such as a painful ear.

Habit spasms (tics)

These abnormal movements or tics tend to affect the older child. They are repetitive, often single, movements which may affect any part such as the face or shoulder and may have their origin, for example, in the blinking of a sore eye. Frequently one particular movement is replaced completely by another habitual movement, e.g. shrugging the shoulder. These movements must be differentiated from chorea, where the movements are non-repetitive and purposeless. The management of tics requires an attempt to discover the psychological causation for the condition and its treatment.

Pica

This abnormality of behaviour may be very severe; the young child may eat such things as sand, stones, coal or other abnormal substances. An iron-deficiency anaemia may be found in some of these patients.

Masturbation

This occurs commonly in children and may be noticed during infancy especially in girls. The thighs may be rubbed together and the infant becomes flushed and resents interference. In the older child the habit may be initiated by some local genital irritation. No treatment is necessary except attracting the child's attention to some other activity.

Breath-holding

Certain young children may hold their breath and become cyanosed, and in extreme cases have a convulsive seizure. These attacks may be initiated by fright or by the child meeting opposition to his desires. The attack may be terminated by inducing an inspiratory movement with cold water or other stimulus.

Reading and writing difficulties

This is a well recognised condition with many differing causes. Mental retardation is an obvious cause and brain damage may be an associated factor; environmental causes may also be important and be related to such factors as overcrowded classes, repeated changes of school and poor home encouragement. Reading and writing difficulty is being recognised in healthy children of normal or superior intelligence and is known as specific dyslexia (and dysgraphia). Boys appear to suffer from dyslexia more often than girls. In their management any specific causal factors should be treated. Children with specific dyslexia require careful management and should be recognised as early as possible so that their progress should not be impeded by their reading problem.

Autism

In 1943 Kanner described autistic children with abnormal behaviour patterns. This group has been widened to include many children with strange and abnormal behaviour. The symptoms usually start early in life; withdrawal symptoms appear and these children are unable to react to their environment in a normal manner. They lack understanding and normal speech is delayed. Some of these patients have normal intelligence. Great difficulty is experienced in their general management. As they grow older they show a gradual improvement and it is important that this improvement be recognised and encouraged. It is essential that special educational facilities be made available for the general management of these children.

The child in hospital

The infant and child is wholly dependent on his mother or a mother substitute from whom he expects to receive security, warmth and physical contact. Up to about the fourth year the child is used to being with his mother for most of the time and he becomes used to a routine and is able to return to his mother for security at certain times. He cannot understand the meaning of illness or separation and is therefore at risk and if at all possible should not be exposed to separation. This separation may allow for the development of behaviour problems and it is essential that paediatric nurses should be understanding and experienced in dealing with these hospital situations where separation has happened. There is little doubt that children in hospital should be visited as much as possible and that visiting should be allowed freely to counteract the emotional effects on the hospitalised child.

17. Mental Subnormality

Mental subnormality is a condition of arrested development of the mind and includes all mentally retarded children from the mildest to the most severe. Intelligence tests are necessary to determine their general management. Special educational requirements are needed for their management; these include special schools (ESN). In the past these mentally subnormal children were divided into the three groups of idiocy, imbecility and feeble-mindedness according to the level of their retardation but these terms are no longer used. They have been replaced with those of subnormality and severe subnormality. Subnormality is a state of arrested or incomplete development of the mind, not amounting to severe subnormality, of a degree requiring medical treatment or other special care or training. Severe subnormality is a state of arrested or incomplete development of the mind, including subnormality of intelligence, of a degree that the patient is incapable of living an independent life or guarding against exploitation.

In order to assess mental retardation it is essential to be aware of the normal milestones of development as discussed in a previous section. Many developmental tests in the infant and young child have been devised and they are of value and are essential in assessing possible cases of mental subnormality and neurological abnormality. There are many antenatal and perinatal factors which are of importance in relation to development. Genetic factors may have an important influence on a child's development and also conditions such as kernicterus will be of significance; this condition is discussed in another section and is an example of an entirely preventable disease. Asphyxia in the perinatal period and neonatal hypoglycaemia are associated with an increasing incidence of late and slow development in the child. Other prenatal and perinatal factors which may be of importance in affecting development in the child include irradiation, certain pregnancy abnormalities such as antepartum haemorrhage, placenta praevia, toxaemia of pregnancy and certain antenatally acquired infections such as toxoplasmosis and cytomegalovirus infection. The best known infection having possible effects on child development is rubella affecting the mother in early pregnancy. Prematurity and low birth weight are of importance and are discussed in another section of this book. Social factors such as poverty and nutrition and the age of the mother are also of importance in relation to an infant's developmental pattern. Environment is undoubtedly of importance in its possible effect on a child's development. There are many diseases and congenital physical abnormalities which are associated with certain degrees of mental subnormality and it is essential that those children who have severe congenital abnormalities have careful assessment of their mental development. Postnatally acquired conditions may also be of importance in affecting intellectual development; these conditions include head injuries and various forms of meningitis and encephalitis. Tuberculous meningitis may be of importance (in affecting mental development especially) where treatment is started at a late stage of the disease. A useful classification to group these conditions is:

1. Primary mental retardation with an intrinsic cause. This group includes such conditions as microcephaly, arrest of development (simple amentia), and Down's syndrome (mongolism).
2. Secondary mental retardation associated with some extrinsic cause. These causes may act:
   (a) antenatally and produce congenital hydrocephalus, porencephaly and spastic diplegia;
   (b) during birth and produce spastic diplegia and other types of cerebral palsy possibly due to anoxic damage at birth;
   (c) postnatal causes, producing the postencephalitic, postmeningitic, hydrocephalic, cretin and traumatic types.

Some of these conditions, such as microcephaly, primary arrest of development and Down's syndrome (mongolism), will be considered in more detail. Other conditions, such as cretinism and hydrocephalus are considered in other sections of this book. Attention is being focused on certain types of mental retardation associated with inborn errors of metabolism; these include the diseases of galactosaemia and phenylketonuria (PKU) and are considered later in this chapter. There are many other rare diseases due to inborn errors of metabolism such as maple syrup urine disease, histidinaemia (which may give a false-positive Phenistix test), Hartnup disease and citrullinuria; no doubt further progress in this field of biochemistry will be made in the future which will allow for better management of these patients.

Microcephaly

True microcephaly is a form of mental deficiency associated with a small head, which is actually due to the small brain. These patients are usually extremely difficult to manage and often require institutional care for their proper management. They are spiteful children and have a very low grade of intelligence. Microcephaly may also be caused by the rare cytomegalovirus infection (Figs 17.1 to 17.3) and by rubella in early pregnancy.

Primary arrest of development

These patients may be slightly below normal in their physical development and have various grades of mental subnormality. This

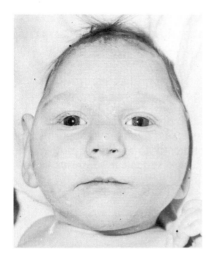

Fig. 17.1 Microcephaly associated with cytomegalic inclusion body disease. The child also had intracranial calcification and chorioretinitis.

Fig. 17.2 Chorioretinitis seen by ophthalmoscopic examination of the fundus of the eye in cytomegalic inclusion body disease (due to cytomegalovirus infection).

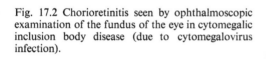

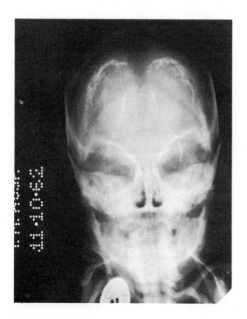

Fig. 17.3 X-ray of skull showing cerebral calcification in cytomegalovirus infection.

retardation may be manifested by very slow development in reaching the various milestones and in their subsequent mental growth. Convulsions may also occur.

Down's syndrome (mongolism) (Figs 17.4 and 17.5)

This condition is unfortunately fairly common. These individuals are always mentally subnormal. The basic cause is unknown, but this type of child is found to be born most frequently to an elderly mother who has had previous normal children; this statement, however, is not

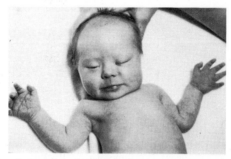

Fig. 17.4 Down's syndrome (mongolism).

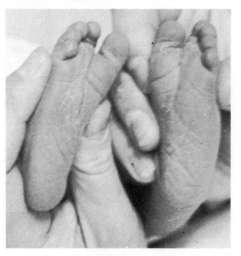

Fig. 17.5 Typical foot of mongol showing the deep cleft between the first and second toes.

absolutely true as frequently they have been born to young mothers as first children. It has been established that these individuals have a chromosomal aberration in that they have 47 chromosomes instead of the normal 46; this appears to be due to a triplication (trisomy) of a small autosomal chromosome (no. 21, or trisomy G—see Fig. 5.42). This disease was first described by Langdon Down in 1866 and is named Down's syndrome.

The diagnosis of Down's syndrome may be made at birth when the facial appearance is the most important feature in recognising the condition. The eyes slant upwards and outwards and have a marked epicanthic fold; if they are blue, small whitish specks and dots (Brushfield's spots) may be seen in the iris encircling the eye at a point in the iris near the corneal margin; these spots, however, are occasionally found in the normal blue-eyed individual. The head is small and may have a flat occiput (brachycephaly). The nostrils are small and the infant often has 'snuffles'. The infant with Down's syndrome tends to protrude the tongue from the mouth, a habit due to a foreshortened jaw and not to a large tongue. The tongue becomes markedly fissured after the age of about 4 years. These individuals have hypotonia and feel very 'floppy'. The hand may show a shortened, inwardly curved fifth finger which on X-ray examination shows a small hypoplastic middle phalanx. The palmar creases may be abnormal showing only a single transverse crease and a marked irregular criss-crossing of other minor creases; the triradiate angle of the palmar print is almost always over 60° in the patient with Down's syndrome, being usually a more acute angle in the normal individual. The foot may show a deep cleft between the first and second toes. A high proportion have congenital heart disease as an additional abnormality and some also have other anomalies such as congenital duodenal obstruction; the incidence of leukaemia appears to be higher in these children. Patients with Down's syndrome are always mentally subnormal but are easily managed children. Their management, whether at home or institutional, depends on the circumstances of each case in relation to the family in which they occur and the availability of a proper institution.

The risk of a second child with Down's syndrome being born to a family is extremely small, although such cases have been recorded. The risk appears to be higher in those that have the rare chromosomal aberration of translocation rather than the more common trisomy abnormality. This is discussed in the section on the chromosomes elsewhere in this book. The differential diagnosis of Down's syndrome (mongolism) is from cretinism, although there is seldom any need to mistake these two conditions. In Down's syndrome the condition can be diagnosed at birth by the typical mongoloid facies and other characteristic features, whereas cretinism can usually be recognised only at 2 to 3 months of age. The cretin has ugly facial features, is pale, has a large tongue, short fingers, dry thickened skin, supraclavicular pads of fat and is very constipated; on the other hand the infant with Down's syndrome has a pink complexion, small protruding tongue (fissured from the age of about 4 years), typical abnormalities of the hands, a soft skin, no supraclavicular pads of fat, has normal bowel function and has a chromosomal abnormality. Furthermore the cretin responds to treatment (thyroid extract) but the child with Down's syndrome does not.

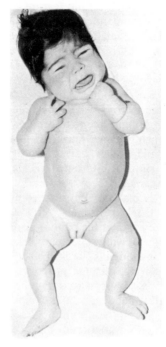

Fig. 17.6 Cretin aged 4 months. (*By courtesy of Dr S. Heymann.*)

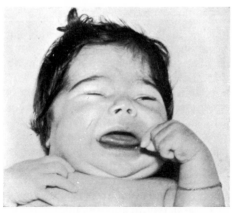

Fig. 17.7 The same infant; note the large tongue. (*By courtesy of Dr S. Heymann.*)

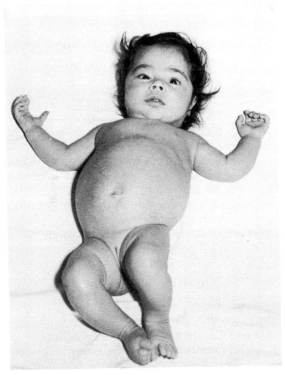

Fig. 17.8 The same infant (Figs 17.6 and 17.7) after some months treatment with thyroid extract.

Metabolic disorders associated with mental subnormality

There are known disorders which are associated with inborn errors of metabolism and mental retardation. Screening methods are available for the early detection of certain of these conditions thereby leading to improved control. These diseases include galactosaemia and phenylketonuria which are discussed in another section of this book.

18. Diseases of the Endocrine System

The endocrine glands produce secretions which are passed directly into the bloodstream. These glands do have an influence on the development of the nervous system and the whole endocrine system is controlled by the hypothalamus. These ductless glands have an important role to perform in relation to the function of the body and are interdependent on each other. Various syndromes may arise in a patient where there is hyperfunction with oversecretion or hypofunction with undersecretion of any particular gland. Some of the different glands will be briefly considered.

THE THYROID GLAND

This endocrine gland develops in the embryo from the primitive foregut and is normally situated in the midline of the neck and lies over the upper part of the trachea. The active principles produced by the thyroid gland are the thyroid hormones which include thyroxine and tri-iodo-thyronine. Approximately one-fifth of the total body iodine is present in the thyroid gland. Thyroxine stimulates metabolism and is also essential for normal growth.

Hyperthyroidism (Graves' disease)

This condition of oversecretion of the thyroid gland is very uncommon in childhood. It is basically the same condition as the adult type and is more common in females. The overactivity in this disease is due to a substance known as 'long-acting thyroid stimulator' (LATS). This substance is one of the globulins associated with IgG and this condition may be due to an autoimmune response to thyroid. In the newborn infant it may affect the baby born of a thyrotoxic mother; this is extremely rare and is a temporary and dangerous condition probably due to the transfer of 'long-acting thyroid stimulator' (LATS) from the mother. It is a self-limited disorder and the 'long-acting thyroid stimulator' may be found in the serum of mother and infant. These infants are very restless and have an agitated appearance and also may have exophthalmos. The skin is warm and flushed and there is marked tachycardia. There may be a slight swelling of the thyroid gland. The treatment of this condition requires that the infant be made euthyroid and the administration of potassium iodide is usually effective.

Thyrotoxicosis in the older child may show the usual symptoms of tachycardia, sweating, exophthalmos, enlargement of the thyroid gland and nervousness. The diagnosis may be confirmed by estimating the protein-bound iodine (PBI) which is raised above the normal range of 4 to 8 μg per cent. Other thyroid tests such as the T_3 and T_4 uptake are also useful in confirming the diagnosis. The treatment requires bed rest and medical treatment should be instituted and this will require the administration of drugs such as carbimazole. Other drugs which are occasionally used are thiouracil of which methylthiouracil is most popular; another drug is potassium perchlorate. The treatment should be continued for a prolonged period of time. Surgical treatment (thyroidectomy) should be delayed if possible until after puberty.

Thyroid swelling (goitre)

In certain districts the thyroid gland may be enlarged from infancy. The swelling is probably associated with a deficiency of iodine and the supply of iodine is necessary in the prevention and treatment of this condition. The swelling may be large enough to produce difficulty in breathing and there may also be evidence of hyposecretion of the gland. Some small goitres may be related to a goitrogenic agent and in these cases the enlargement may be prevented by the administration of iodine. Some sporadic cases are also due to iodine deficiency as in endemic goitre. Sporadic goitre may be controlled in certain cases by iodising salt.

If there are nodules present in the enlarged gland a thyroid scan and possibly a biopsy is necessary to exclude a neoplasm.

Hypothyroidism (Figs. 18.1 to 18.3)

There are various types of hypothyroidism which may occur of which cretinism is the most severe. Other types include juvenile myx-oedema, the accidental ingestion of goitrogenic agents and primary autoimmune thyroiditis such as Hashimoto's disease. Cretinism is associated with a gross lack of thyroid secretion and may occur as a sporadic condition and also in goitrous regions associated with a goitre as endemic cretinism. The disease is not usually recognised at birth but becomes manifest at about the age of 6 to 10 weeks. This is probably related to the infant being maintained in the early postnatal period by maternal secretions. In the neonatal period prolonged jaundice may be present and with this suspicion early diagnosis may be made by thyroid function tests.

The cretin has a number of typical features. The facies usually become coarse and ugly and the skin is dry, firm and cold. The hair tends to be thin and falls out easily. The anterior fontanelle remains open for a longer period than normal and the fingers tend to be short and stumpy. An umbilical hernia is often present and there may be thickened areas of fat present above the clavicles. The tongue is enlarged and protrudes from the mouth. At a later age there is a tendency towards a lumbar lordosis and dorsal kyphosis. The untreated cretin fails to grow and has a short stature. The voice is deep and croaky and the child shows little activity. Constipation becomes severe and feeding difficulties and noisy breathing may be present. Mental subnormality

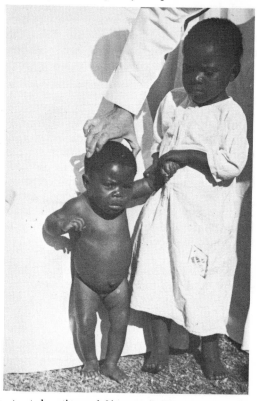

Fig. 18.1 An untreated cretin aged 3½ years (height 65 cm) photographed with a normal child of the same age.

of a severe type is usually present in the untreated case. It is important to confirm the diagnosis as soon as possible so that treatment will not be delayed and it is essential to recognise that in early cases all the described features may not be present. Confirmatory evidence for the diagnosis may be sought by various investigations such as radiology, to detect a delay in bone development and abnormality of the lumbar spine, and also evidence of epiphyseal abnormality, electrocardiography, thyroid function tests including the T_3 and T_4 uptake investigation and thyroxine levels, blood cholesterol levels (often raised in

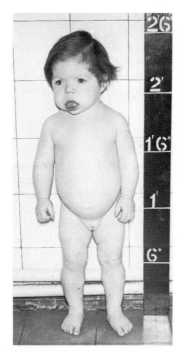

Fig. 18.2 Untreated cretin.

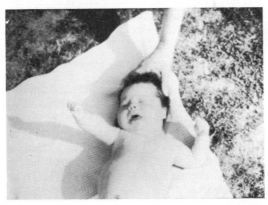

Fig. 18.3 Untreated cretin.

cretinism above the normal of 4·0 to 7·5 mmol per litre), a low alkaline phosphatase, anaemia and a low protein-bound iodine (PBI).

The differential diagnosis from Down's syndrome (mongolism) is often mentioned, but there are few similarities between these two conditions. The main distinguishing features are discussed in the section on Down's syndrome.

Prognosis

The outlook in cretinism depends to a large extent on when treatment is started. The sooner treatment is commenced the better is the outlook regarding normal mental development but this cannot be guaranteed as even with very early treatment there may be associated mental subnormality. Physical development is usually very good when treatment is started early.

Treatment

This requires the administration of thyroid extract in the form of L-thyroxine (Eltroxin) orally. The starting dose should be 0·025 mg (25 μg) of L-thyroxine once daily, gradually increasing the amount to the optimum maximum that the infant will tolerate. A good clinical observation of adequate dosage is one bowel movement daily in addition to an assessment of the general development of the patient. It is important to stress that these patients must take thyroid daily for the life-long period and parents should be warned against discontinuing the therapy.

With this treatment growth will be normal and it is necessary that adequate vitamin D requirements are provided to prevent rickets developing in the growing bones.

Other diseases of the thyroid gland are extremely rare and these include acute inflammatory conditions (acute thyroiditis) and thyroid carcinoma. In this malignant condition the gland is usually nodular and it is essential that a thyroid scan and biopsy be performed to confirm or exclude the possibility of malignancy.

THE PITUITARY GLAND

The pituitary gland is situated at the base of the skull and is extremely important in controlling bodily functions and is also closely related to the proper control of the functions of all the other ductless glands probably related to the hypothalamus. The anterior part of the pituitary gland produces a secretion which has a profound effect on normal growth, and other secretions which affect and control the functions of the other glands. Adrenocorticotrophic hormone (ACTH) is an example and this stimulates the cortex of the adrenal gland to produce cortisone. The posterior pituitary gland secretes pituitrin, which has an important effect on the secretion of urine by acting in the hypothalamic part of the brain. Where there is dysfunction of this part which interferes with the effect of this antidiuretic hormone, the condition of *diabetes insipidus* arises.

In this condition there is profound thirst and this is associated with the passage of large amounts of dilute urine of low specific gravity with the inability to concentrate urine. The condition may be associated with any disease which affects the posterior pituitary and hypothalamic regions; these diseases include basal meningitis, encephalitis, syphilis, trauma to the base of the skull and the rare Hand-Schüller-Christian disease with its xanthomatous deposits.

In Hand-Schüller-Christian disease, apart from the diabetes insipidus, there may be associated splenomegaly and exophthalmos. Pitressin may be of benefit in controlling the excessive diuresis and is available as an injection of pitressin tannate or as a snuff or a nasal spray in the form of lysine vasopressin (lypressin). The polyuria may also be controlled by the administration of chlorothiazide. The primary disease should if possible be treated.

Different types of short stature may be associated with hyposecretion of the anterior pituitary gland. In these cases human growth hormone may be administered but deficiency of this hormone must be demonstrated, for which the 'Bovril' test may be useful. The condition of Frohlich's syndrome or dystrophia adiposogenitalis is associated with small stature, obesity, hypoplasia of the genitalia and may be due to a tumour in the neighbourhood of the pituitary gland affecting the secretion.

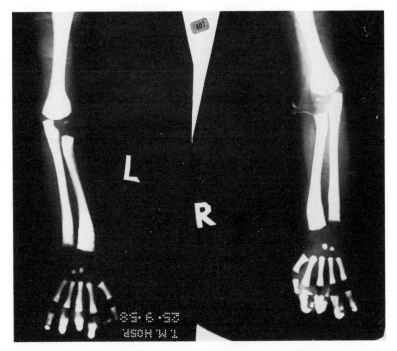

Fig. 18.4 X-ray of upper limbs in Albers-Schönberg disease ('marble bones').

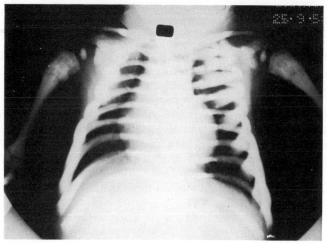

Fig. 18.5 X-ray of chest in Albers-Schönberg disease showing sclerosis of bones (osteopetrosis—'marble bones').

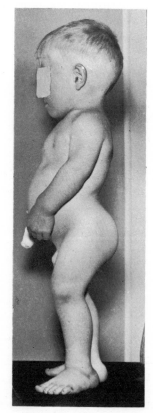

Fig. 18.6 Photograph of a male child of 7 years of short stature measuring 82·5 cm in height. Note the lumbar lordosis and short limbs. This patient suffers from a type of chondrodystrophy.

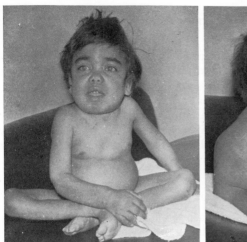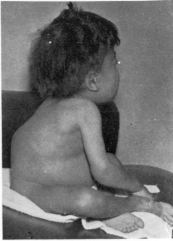

Fig. 18.7 A child suffering from gargoylism. Age 7 years. This patient is of short stature and has other disabilities. Note the corneal cloudiness of both eyes and the typical facies.

Fig. 18.8 A lateral photograph of the same patient as in previous figure showing the marked spinal kyphosis.

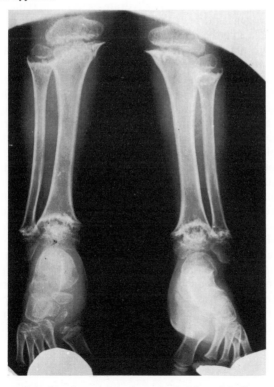

Fig. 18.9 X-ray of the long bones of the lower leg in Morquio's disease showing the irregularity of the epiphyses.

Hypersecretion of the anterior pituitary gland in childhood produces an overgrowth of the skeleton with the condition of gigantism. This condition may be associated with a tumour of the eosinophil cells of the anterior pituitary gland (adenoma). The basophil cells of the anterior pituitary may also produce a small tumour but the symptoms of gross obesity, striae of the skin and hypertension (Cushing's syndrome) is due to hyperaction of the adrenal cortex although a central cause may lie in the hypothalamus.

THE ADRENAL GLAND

There are two adrenal glands each situated on the upper pole of a kidney. In the newborn infant they are very large, rapidly becoming smaller, due to atrophy of a part of the cortex of the gland. The adrenal gland is made up of two distinct parts, which differ in origin, development and function. These parts are the medulla and the cortex. The medulla produces adrenalin with its important bodily function. The cortex produces hormones which control water and electrolyte metabolism (mineralocorticoids), carbohydrate metabolism (glucocorticoids) and the androgens and oestrogens controlling sex function.

The medulla may be affected by neoplasms such as neuroblastoma and phaeochromocytoma. The neuroblastoma is a malignant tumour which tends to spread to the liver (Pepper's tumour) or to the orbit and skull (Hutchison's tumour) and the long bones. These may be secreting tumours and a useful test for this secretion is to estimate the vanillylmandelic acid (VMA) secretion in the urine. In the treatment of this condition, apart from the use of surgery and radiation therapy in the few early localised cases, chemotherapy should be used in the form of cyclophosphamide or vincristine.

A phaeochromocytoma is a rare tumour of the medulla which produces an adrenalin substance (noradrenalin) and gives rise to attacks of hypertension with headache and sweating. This tumour may be successfully removed with a complete cure of the condition. An essential test in diagnosis of this condition is the estimation of the urinary VMA excretion which reflects the catecholamine level.

The cortex may rarely be affected by a benign or malignant tumour or hypertrophy with overproduction of the hormones of this part of the adrenal gland. As mentioned, this excessive production of secretion may give rise to differing syndromes such as Cushing's (hypertension, hirsutism and obesity) or the adrenogenital syndrome with intersex or sexual precocity.

19. Some Surgical and Orthopaedic Conditions of Infancy and Childhood

The infant and child may be affected by numerous surgical and ortho-paedic disorders both rare and common (Figs 19.1 to 19.12). Brief consideration will be given to some of these disorders.

Harelip and cleft-palate (Fig. 19.4)

These are congenital abnormalities of development and may exist together or separately. There are various types of this disorder depending upon the extent of the abnormality of development in a failure of fusion of the various parts of the face and palate. Diagnosis is made on inspection of the infant after birth. Difficulty may be experienced in feeding the child; however, with patience, many of these infants may even be fed efficiently on the breast; if this is impossible, then success may be obtained by bottle or spoonfeeding. The treatment requires expert surgical repair by a plastic surgeon. The lip is repaired when the child has reached a weight of 4·5 kg and is clinically well. The palate should be repaired later, at any time before speech has started. A dental prosthesis can be made for the palate soon after birth; this may be extremely useful in the management of these infants. An uncommon abnormality of micrognathos often with a cleft-palate and the tendency for the tongue to fall backwards into the pharynx (glossoptosis) some-times occurs. This is known as the Pierre-Robin syndrome (Fig. 5.3) and requires careful nursing and positional care in early infancy to prevent the tongue falling backwards into the pharynx and thereby asphyxiating the child. On occasions, surgical interference is necessary to fix the tongue forward.

Congenital atresia of the bowel (Fig. 19.6)

With small bowel atresia, often affecting the duodenum, the newborn infant starts vomiting soon after birth. X-ray examination is essential in confirming the diagnosis and urgent surgical relief of the intestinal obstruction is necessary to save life. Unfortunately these atresias of the bowel are often multiple. Congenital abnormalities of the oesophagus have been considered in another section. An imperforate anus (Fig. 19.7) is easily diagnosed by careful routine examination of every newly born infant; if present, surgical relief is essential.

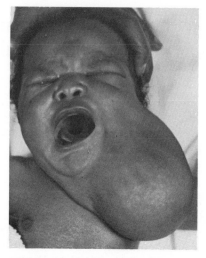

Fig. 19.1 Large cystic hygroma of the neck.

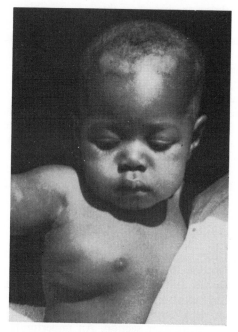

Fig. 19.2 Large benign lipomatous tumour in an infant.

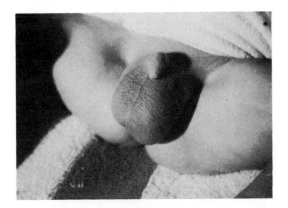

Fig. 19.3 Scrotal swelling due to a hydrocele.

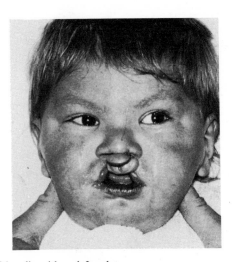

Fig. 19.4 Bilateral harelip with a cleft-palate.

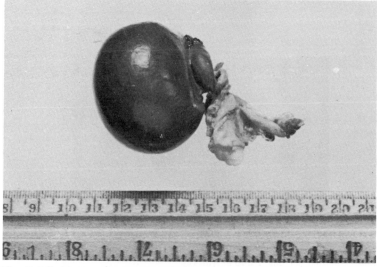

Fig. 19.5 Twisted ovarian cyst in an infant.

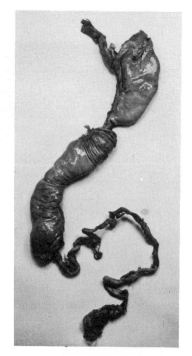

Fig. 19.6 Specimen showing congenital atresia of the bowel.

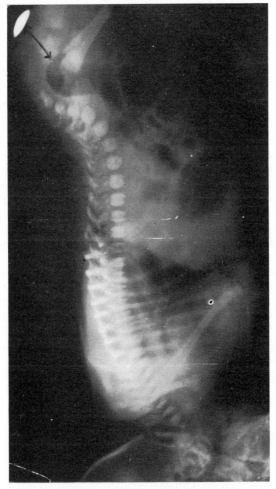

Fig. 19.7 Radiograph of a newborn infant with an imperforate anus taken upside down to show the distance between the rectum and the skin marked with a radio-opaque metal marker.

Hirschsprung's disease

This rare condition, commoner in boys, gives rise to a clinical picture of extreme constipation and abdominal distension with dilatation of the colon. The cause of the condition has been clearly described; it is due to an absence of nerve ganglia and nerve plexus in a segment of the sigmoid colon which prevents the normal functioning of that part of the bowel, with consequent obstruction and extreme constipation. Treatment requires the surgical excision of the deficient segment of bowel with anastomosis above and below the resected portion (Swensen's operation) or the Duhamel operation.

Intussusception

This condition is not uncommon and is very dramatic in its onset; it is dangerous to life if not treated urgently. The condition affects male infants more frequently than females; the commonest age-group affected is 6 to 18 months and the child is usually previously well. The condition is due to the invagination of part of the bowel (usually terminal ileum) into the more distal part of the bowel (usually colon). The invaginating portion is called the intussusceptum. If not relieved this condition gives rise to intestinal obstruction and gangrene of the invaginated portion of bowel.

The clinical picture is one of acute sudden episodes of abdominal pain with the child drawing up his legs, screaming and becoming pale and exhausted. These attacks are repeated, and eventually the infant passes a stool of bright red blood and mucus (red-currant jelly stool). Vomiting occurs and if the condition is not relieved the child becomes extremely ill and toxic. The intussusception may be felt on abdominal examination as a sausage-shaped tumour, and may eventually, in rare cases, even present at the anus. The general measures to relieve dehydration and toxaemia with intravenous therapy are essential, and urgent surgical operation and reduction of the intussusception is necessary.

Acute appendicitis

This is the commonest cause of an acute abdomen in childhood. The symptomatology includes vomiting and pain in the abdomen; constipation is often present although diarrhoea may occur with a pelvic appendicitis. Pyrexia and a rising pulse rate are important features in this disease. Abdominal tenderness in the right iliac fossa, with muscle guarding and rigidity, is found on examination. The white blood cells are usually raised (leucocytosis). This condition requires urgent surgical intervention and removal of the appendix, if perforation with the development of dangerous peritonitis is to be avoided. The differential diagnosis of a case of acute appendicitis is, amongst other conditions, from the condition of mesenteric adenitis.

Pneumococcal peritonitis

This condition usually affects girls and may follow an attack of vulvovaginitis spreading to the peritoneum. Abdominal pain, pyrexia and vomiting are often found and there may be difficulty in differentiating the condition from acute appendicitis. The treatment is conservative and requires expert nursing in modified Fowler's position with the use of antibiotics and chemotherapy in adequate dosage.

Rectal prolapse

In this condition the mucosa of the rectum prolapses downwards producing a reddish swollen mass at the anus, with a tendency to bleed. It tends to occur in debilitated children and may be associated with a diarrhoeal disorder or with constipation and it is also found on occasions in children with cystic fibrosis (fibrocystic disease of the pancreas, mucoviscidosis). Treatment of this condition requires replacement of the prolapsed mucosa and strapping the buttocks with plaster to prevent recurrence. General treatment of debility is essential as is also the proper management of any associated disease.

Curvature of the spine

These postural defects are common in childhood and may take the form of scoliosis (lateral curvature), kyphosis (anteroposterior curvature) or lordosis (excessive curvature in the lumbar region). These defects often affect poorly developed children with bad posture; correct training and exercises are useful in their management.

Congenital dislocation of the hip

This is a congenital abnormality present from birth. Females are affected more commonly than males and it is seen more often after a breech delivery; it also appears to be more common on the left side than the right although both hips may be affected and it may also have a familial tendency. All newborn infants should be specially examined to detect the possible presence of this condition so that treatment can be instituted as early as possible. In the neonatal screening for this condition Barlow's modification of Ortolani's test is used. Diagnostic signs in the affected hip in the newborn infant are the restriction of abduction and the presence of a 'click' on abducting the flexed hip. Walking may be delayed. In the untreated case a bilateral condition gives rise to a waddling gait. Radiological examination is essential in confirming the diagnosis. The sooner treatment is started, the better the prognosis. It requires prolonged positioning of the lower limbs in a position of abduction with flexed knees and the von Rosen splint is extremely useful for this purpose in the very young infant.

Club-foot (talipes equinovarus) (Fig. 19.8)

This congenital abnormality is easily diagnosed at birth. With efficient treatment the outlook for these cases is good. Treatment requires manipulation and splintage to correct the deformities.

Congenital enlargement of the toe may be effectively treated by surgery (Fig. 19.9).

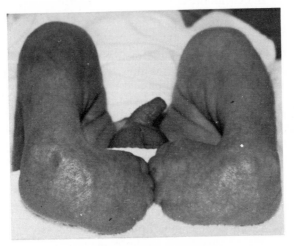

Fig. 19.8 Bilateral club-feet (talipes equinovarus).

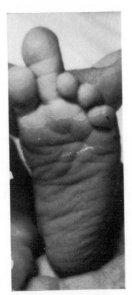

Fig. 19.9 Congenital enlargement of the second toe (left) in a newborn infant.

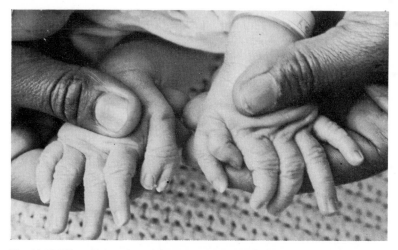

Fig. 19.10 Bilateral preaxial polydactyly showing double thumbs.

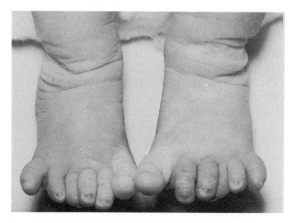

Fig. 19.11 Bilateral polydactyly.

Perthes' disease

This disease of epiphyseal abnormality is due to osteochondritis affecting the hip joint. It affects males more commonly than females and usually starts between the fifth and tenth years. The main complaint of the child is a limp later followed by pain in the hip. X-ray examination of the affected joint shows the typical flattening followed by fragmentation of the head of the femur. Treatment requires prolonged rest of the affected joint using a weight-bearing caliper or a 'broomstick' plaster.

Tuberculosis of the spine

Tuberculosis of bone and joint has become rare in countries where there has been a reduction in the incidence of tuberculosis.

Tuberculous affection of the spine most commonly affects the thoracic vertebrae; the clinical features vary and these patients may complain of pain, especially on bending. The spinal muscles develop spasm and the patient will not bend his back, e.g. to pick up an object from the ground. X-ray examination is essential in the diagnosis and control of such a case; the vertebral body is affected with eventual collapse. Treatment requires absolute rest in a plaster bed for a very long term. Antituberculosis drugs are necessary in the treatment, in addition to the general measures usually adopted in chronic tuberculous patients.

Tuberculosis of the hip joint

The hip is the commonest joint to be affected by tuberculosis. The child complains of pain in the joint and it is associated with a limp. The limb shows limitation in movement in all directions and X-ray examination is essential. The Mantoux reaction is positive in most cases of joint and bone tuberculosis. The treatment requires prolonged immobilisation of the affected limb together with the use of the antituberculosis drugs such as isoniazid (INAH), rifampicin and sodium amino-salicylate; in addition to these measures the general principles of treatment such as good nursing, good nourishing food, fresh air and sunshine are necessary.

The knee is another joint commonly affected by tuberculosis. The therapeutic measures are similar to those in hip joint disease.

Child abuse ('battered baby' syndrome) (Fig. 19.12)

This syndrome is being recognised as a condition where symptoms and signs occur in children, usually under 2 years of age, who have suffered repeated physical maltreatment and injury at the hands of parents or others. Although the majority of injuries to small children are accidental it is necessary to be aware that such injury may have maltreatment as the cause. Small children with fractures, bruising, repeated injuries or swellings should alert the observer to the possibility of this syndrome. In the clinical investigation of these cases radiological examination for bone injury is essential. It should be recognised that the occurrence of this condition is an indication of some serious underlying family disturbance and the management of this serious problem requires the team co-operation of the family doctor, the health

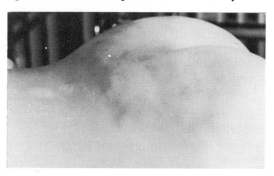

Fig. 19.12 Non-accidental injury in childhood. (Child abuse—'battered baby' syndrome.)

visitor, the paediatrician, the social worker and most important of all the overall control of the Social Service Department of the Local Authority. Unfortunately it is usually impossible to anticipate the first episode of maltreatment but there is little doubt that early diagnosis is an extremely important part of future prevention. The parents require supportive treatment with the use of social and psychiatric assistance so that the child may be protected from future injury.

Burns

Burns and scalds are common happenings in childhood. The degree of accompanying shock is directly related to the area involved and is associated with haemoconcentration. All children with burns affecting over 10 per cent of the total surface area require urgent treatment. The surface area affected in children over 10 years of age can be calculated by using the rule of 'nines'; in smaller children the head is proportionately larger and at birth accounts for 19 per cent of the surface area so that allowance must be made for this in calculating the surface area involved. Treatment requires intravenous therapy with plasma or blood and dextrose saline solutions to replace fluid loss and for maintenance of fluid requirements. Closed or open exposed methods of treatment are used and it is necessary that infection be controlled and skin grafting can be useful. Lyophilised cadaveric skin preparations are available to provide temporary protective covering for burned areas which are later covered by homografts.

20. Diseases of the Skin

Protection from trauma and infection is an important function of the skin. In addition, there are the normal secretory functions of the sweat and sebaceous glands of the skin and also the temperature regulatory function. A certain amount of absorption of different substances by the skin can also occur.

Affections of the skin may be classified as follows:

1. Congenital abnormalities
2. Acquired affections in the newborn
3. Infections and infestations (dermatitis)—bacterial, viral, fungal and parasitic
4. Allergic conditions
5. Toxic conditions
6. Exanthemata
7. Neoplasms
8. Miscellaneous conditions

The following terms are used for describing various eruptions of the skin:

A *macular* eruption is a discoloration, often red or pinkish in colour, which is not raised above the skin surface. An example of this type occurs in some of the infectious fevers.

A *papular* eruption is similar to the macular type except that it is raised above the level of the skin. An example is the eruption of measles.

A *vesicular* eruption is small raised lesions of the skin with some clear fluid in them. This type occurs in chickenpox.

A *bullous* eruption is similar to the vesicular type except that the affected areas are larger.

A *pustular* eruption is the same as the vesicular variety, but the lesions contain pus. This occurs in smallpox.

A *petechial* lesion is one associated with a small amount of extravasated blood in the skin such as occurs in purpura.

Congenital abnormalities

These conditions include the disease of ichthyosis (Figs 20.1 and 20.2) and ichthyosiform conditions where the skin is dry and scaly and thickened keratinised changes occur. The most extreme form of this condition is the Harlequin foetus which is incompatible with survival longer than a few days. Many of these ichthyoṣiform conditions are hereditary and some may be transmitted as an autosomal recessive where the risk of a similar condition occurring in a sibling is one in four. The mild type of ichthyosis may be called xeroderma. In these conditions of hyperkeratosis one of the main problems is the lack of water-binding substance in the horny layer of the skin where the dryness and scaliness occurs. A useful preparation in the treatment of these condi-

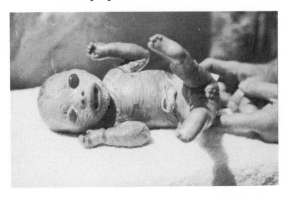

Fig. 20.1 Harlequin foetus (congenital ichthyosis). Note the marked skin abnormality with cracks and fissures and also the eversion of the eyelids. (*By courtesy of Dr S. N. Javett.*)

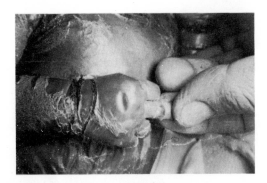

Fig. 20.2 Collodion skin; a form of ichthyosis.

tions is the local application of a urea substance, carbamide (Calmurid). This substance appears to assist in retaining water in the skin by increasing the concentration of water-binding substances in the skin. A very uncommon congenital abnormality is epidermolysis bullosa; this condition is associated with the production of blisters or bullae on any part of the skin subjected to trauma. Another extremely rare congenital abnormality of the skin is incontinentia pigmenti (Bloch-

Sulzberger syndrome (Fig. 20.3) which appears to affect only females and is associated with the early development at birth or soon after, of blisters on the limbs and trunk. The lesions eventually subside leaving pigmentary abnormality in the areas affected in the form of whorls and linear lesions; this condition may be associated with other abnormalities affecting the eyes, hair and teeth. Commoner congenital abnormalities of the skin are the naevi. There are different varieties of this condition,

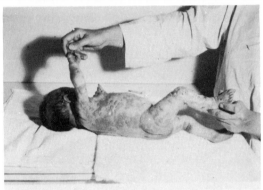

Fig. 20.3 Incontinentia pigmenti (Bloch-Sulzberger syndrome).

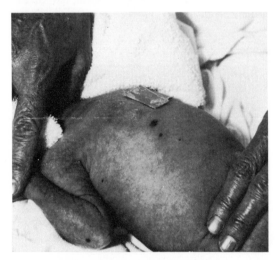

Fig. 20.4 Newborn infant with multiple haemangiomata.

all of which are types of haemangiomata (Figs 20.4, 20.5 and 20.6). The 'port-wine' mark occurs on any part of the body and is a flat lesion. A similar haemangioma may be present on the forehead on one or other side in a position in relation to the distribution of the ophthalmic branch of the trigeminal (5th cranial) nerve. This lesion may be associated with a haemangioma of the brain which may cause fits and may become calcified (Sturge-Weber syndrome). The 'strawberry mark' is a small raised lesion, reddish in colour, which may extend into the sub-

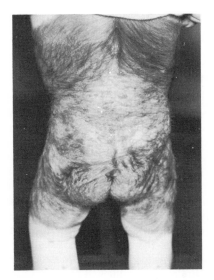

Fig. 20.5 Extensive pigmented naevus.

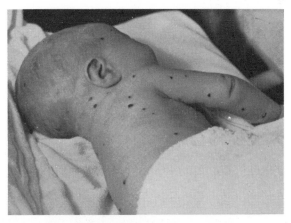

Fig. 20.6 An unusual skin disease in the newborn resembling a naevoxanthoendothelioma. (*By courtesy from Kessel, Van Dongen & Proctor: 'Journal of Obstetrics and Gynaecology of the British Commonwealth'*.)

cutaneous tissue as a capillary cavernous naevus; these capillary cavernous haemangiomata usually disappear spontaneously in later life. In childhood they may be treated by surgery.

Acquired affections in the newborn

The conditions of pemphigus neonatorum and Ritter's disease have been considered in the section on the newborn.

Infections and infestations

Bacterial. The skin may be infected with the staphylococcal organism and produce a crusted, weeping eruption, usually affecting the face; this condition can also be caused by a haemolytic streptococcus and is known as impetigo contagiosum. The first essential in treatment is to remove the crusts, after which an antibiotic preparation may be applied. The haemolytic streptococcus as a cause may on rare occasions be complicated by the development of sensitisation reactions such as nephritis as discussed in another section. Tuberculosis of the skin is extremely rare in childhood but it may occur secondary to the breaking down of a tuberculous cervical gland or as the primary condition of lupus vulgaris. In lupus the skin lesions usually begin as numerous small disseminated or grouped flat papules which gradually enlarge to form the typical apple-jelly nodules. This disease is very chronic and requires the usual antituberculosis treatment in addition to the general principles of fresh air and an adequate diet. The skin manifestations of congenital syphilis are considered in Chapter 21.

Viral (Fig. 20.7). The virus of herpes simplex (*Herpesvirus hominis*)

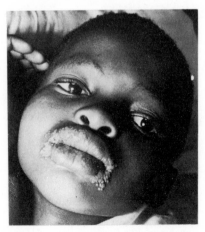

Fig. 20.7 Herpes labialis in a patient with meningococcal meningitis.

produces the 'fever blister' (herpes febrilis or labialis) around the mouth and nostrils associated with cases of the common cold, meningococcal meningitis and pneumonia. This herpesvirus may also produce a stomatitis as discussed in another section of this book.

Herpes zoster (shingles) is also a virus infection affecting the posterior nerve root ganglion and producing the segmental painful vesicular lesions of the skin (Fig. 20.8) which run along the course of a nerve. Local application of an idoxuridine solution in dimethylsulphoxide (Herpid) may be useful. This is an uncommon condition in childhood, but it is interesting to note that where cases of herpes zoster occur in a household, for example, the contacts may develop chickenpox; the same virus causes these two diseases.

Another virus is the cause of molluscum contagiosum where small benign swellings of the skin occur in the young child; they have a characteristic waxy appearance with central umbilication. They may be

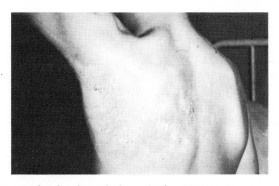

Fig. 20.8 Herpes zoster showing the vesicular and crusted lesions along the course of a thoracic nerve.

found on any part of the skin and may disappear spontaneously in association with an inflammatory reaction. The treatment requires that the lesion be shelled out with a sharp instrument and phenol probed into the lesion.

Verrucae, or the common wart, is due to a virus infection which produces the well-known skin lesion found so often in children. The common wart is a raised lesion with a pitted surface and is commonly found on the fingers and hands but may occur on any part of the skin. The plantar wart is usually flat on account of pressure and is usually painful; multiple warts are not uncommon. Other types of warts occur such as the filiform type with fine projections and a keratinised tip. These, however, are more frequently found in the adult. Verrucae are contagious and may be difficult to dislodge. Single lesions may be treated with a chemical caustic substance or an electric cautery.

Fungal. Ringworm or tinea affections are common in childhood and are caused by fungi. They may affect the body, the hairy scalp or the nails. They are contagious conditions and are caused by the following fungi: the microsporon, the trichophyton and the epidermophyton. Tinea capitis or ringworm of the scalp is often caused by the *Microsporon audouini* or uncommonly by a trichophyton. A small scaly patch appears on the scalp with thinning of the hair, and this may be followed by other affected patches. An affected hair may be removed and examined in liq. potass.; the typical appearance, microscopically, of a mosaic sheath may be seen.

Tinea corporis, or ringworm of the non-hairy skin, may occur in different types, the circinate type being commonest; this appears as roundish, scaly patches or rings on the face, trunk or extremities. It may be caused by the microsporon or trichophyton. The scales may be examined microscopically to show the fungus. This type responds very well to the application of different antifungal remedies such as Whitfield's ointment, brilliant green paint or tincture of iodine. Ringworm of the nails is very uncommon and produces thickening of the nail bed. Favus is another fungal condition of the skin producing thickened rounded affected areas with scarring, often appearing on the scalp.

An antibiotic, griseofulvin, fine particle (Grisovin, Fulcin) is available for the treatment of difficult resistant cases of these fungal infections of the skin, scalp or nails; this drug is administered by mouth and usually has very gratifying results.

Parasitic. Pediculosis is due to lice, and three types may affect man: *Pediculosis capitis, Pediculosis corporis* and *Pediculosis pubis.* They occur in children who lack proper care and live in poor hygienic surroundings. The eggs, or 'nits', are found firmly attached to individual hairs and there is difficulty in removing them. The infected person scratches the affected part and secondary infection frequently occurs. Thorough washing, with the application of an antiparasitic preparation such as dicophane or gamma benzene hexachloride and subsequent combing should be used as therapy.

Scabies is a condition due to the itch-mite *Acarus* or *Sarcoptes scabiei* and also affects children who lack proper care. The chief lesion is a burrow in the skin affecting mainly the fingers. This is associated with extreme itchiness, especially at night when the patient is in bed. The condition is contagious. The most satisfactory treatment is the application of a 25 per cent benzyl benzoate emulsion (Ascabiol) following a hot bath with thorough washing. This treatment may be repeated and associated with this treatment the clothing and bed clothing must be adequately sterilised to remove any infestation which would allow for the reinfestation of the patient. Gamma benzene hexachloride lotion or cream (Quellada, Lorexane, Esoderm) is also effective in the treatment of scabies.

Allergic conditions

Infantile eczema (*atopic dermatitis*) (Fig. 20.9). This is a common condition which affects fair-skinned children and usually occurs after the third month. The face is first affected with a reddish, irritating lesion which tends to spread. The lesion may be moist and is very irritating, leading to much scratching with aggravation of the affected parts. The rest of the body may be affected and the lesions may dry and become flaky. These infants may develop acute diarrhoeal disorders of a severe type. Irritation of the affected parts by scratching or contact with rough clothing tends to aggravate the condition and also introduce secondary infection. Certain foods such as cow's milk or eggs may intensify the lesions. The ultimate prognosis is good and the condition, although very protracted, eventually clears up; the older child, however, may develop a dermatitis affecting the flexural surfaces, such as those at the elbow, the knee or the neck, with thickened, itchy, eczematous areas of

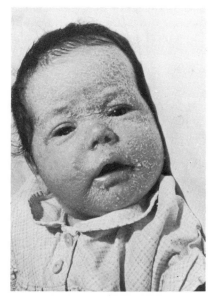

Fig. 20.9 Infantile eczema.

skin being present (Besnier's prurigo or flexural eczema). There is often a family history of allergy in these patients and in later life the patient may develop other allergic conditions.

Treatment of infantile eczema includes

1. The protection of the skin from irritation by preventing scratching; therapeutic agents such as trimeprazine (Vallergan) are useful.

2. The application of some bland preparation such as a crude coal tar ointment in the quiescent phase or a zinc cream in the active red phase are helpful.
3. The use of antibiotics to treat secondary infection.
4. Dietetic measures in an attempt to remove the causative agent if known.
5. Corticosteroid therapy is very useful in the acute phase and the local application of one per cent hydrocortisone ointment gives relief as may other topical corticosteroid preparations.

Urticaria. This may occur in childhood as a papular urticaria; it starts as a papular lesion which may become vesicular and affects mainly the lower limbs, the buttocks or the trunk. The lesions may be very itchy. It is thought that this condition is usually associated with insect bites such as those of fleas or bugs. The prognosis is excellent as it tends to disappear as the child grows up. True urticaria also frequently occurs in childhood as the typical itchy weal. It may be caused by various agents such as strawberries or as a manifestation of serum sickness. The antihistamine drugs are useful in treating this condition in addition to a soothing local application such as calamine lotion.

Toxic conditions

Drugs. Some drugs such as aspirin, penicillin, barbiturates or the sulphonamide preparations may produce a variety of eruptions ranging from erythematous lesions to the purpuric types. Certain drugs, however, may produce a specific type of eruption. Bromides may produce an acniform or papular eruption of the face. The belladonna group of drugs may produce a reddish flush of the skin in addition to other toxic manifestations. A soap and water enema may produce an erythematous rash about 12 hours later.

The exanthemata

The different acute infectious fevers such as rubella, measles, chicken-pox, smallpox and scarlet fever all have their distinctive rashes; these will be discussed in a later section.

Neoplasms

Malignant conditions of the skin are extremely rare in childhood. Adenoma sebaceum may occur in children as reddish papules on the face; it may be associated with fits and mental retardation in the condition known as tuberose sclerosis (epiloia) (Fig. 20.10).

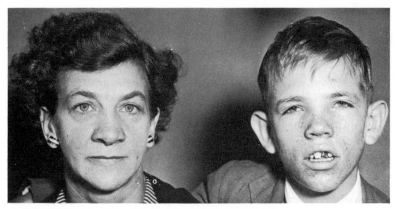

Fig. 20.10 Tuberose sclerosis (epiloia) in mother and son.

Miscellaneous conditions

Erythema nodosum (Fig. 20.11). This is a condition usually occurring as multiple, oval-shaped, reddish lesions most commonly on the legs along the tibial bone. They go through the colour changes of a bruise, becoming purplish and then fading completely leaving a slight stain of the skin. The condition is due to a sensitivity reaction of the patient,

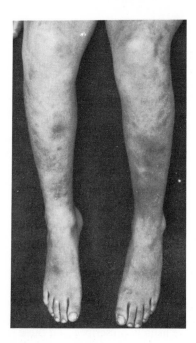

Fig. 20.11 Lesions of erythema nodosum.

usually to some infection such as tuberculosis or a streptococcal infection. In these cases it is always important to investigate the patient for a tuberculous infection. Ingestion of sulphathiazole has also led to the development of erythema nodosum.

Napkin rash. Infants who have diarrhoea may develop a reddish, angry-looking lesion of the buttocks affecting those parts in contact with the wet napkin. The lesion is in the nature of a burn and is probably due to the effect of faecal organisms on urine, producing excessive ammonia with the development of an ammoniacal burn. Proper cleanliness and sterilisation of napkins, together with a bland application to the rash (zinc and castor oil cream) is necessary to heal the condition. Monilia infection of the buttocks has been referred to in a previous section.

Sclerema neonatorum. This rare condition affects the newborn infant and produces a peculiar thickening of the subcutaneous tissues. It may affect the premature infant and may become generalised. ACTH and corticosteroid therapy may be of some value in this serious disease.

Psoriasis (Fig. 20.12). This is a chronic skin disease and may occur in childhood. The main lesion in this condition is a scaly papule which may coalesce to form multiple lesions; they usually affect the whole

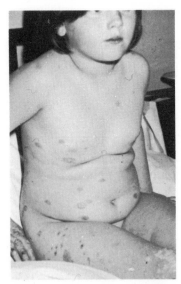

Fig. 20.12 Psoriasis in a child. Note the lesions on the trunk, thigh and hand.

body including the scalp. The cause of this disease is unknown although it may be hereditary and may be transmitted as a dominant condition. Local applications are usually prescribed and these include tar preparations. Natural sunshine and dithranol may be helpful.

21. Acute Infectious and Contagious Fevers

Rubella (German measles)

This is a very common infectious disease which affects individuals of any age but usually children. It is due to a virus and has an incubation period of 14 to 21 days; the virus has been isolated and identified. The disease is relatively mild and is characterised by a slight pyrexia, a macular rash which lasts about two days and enlargement of the cervical and occipital lymph glands. There is no specific treatment. Much attention has been focused on this disease in relation to its occurrence in women in early pregnancy and this aspect is the most significant part of this virus infection. It has been definitely established that the foetus of such a pregnancy may be severely harmed in relation to the production of congenital anomalies (affecting mainly the heart, brain, eyes or ears). Apart from the congenital anomalies that may be produced by rubella the foetus may also be born with evidence of widespread infection; purpura might be present and also thrombocytopenia (reduction of platelets), hepatomegaly, splenomegaly and certain bone lesions detected by X-ray. The newborn infant with congenital rubella may be a source of infection to contacts as the virus may still be present and passed for many weeks. With the isolation and identification of the virus of rubella a vaccine is available for use in initiating active immunisation of females, thereby controlling and preventing this important cause of congenital abnormality. The preparation available is a live attenuated rubella virus vaccine (Almevax, Cendevax) and a single dose appears to be sufficient to induce immunity. The principal aim of using this vaccine is to obtain immunity in women before pregnancy thereby preventing the rubella syndrome in the newborn. It is preferable that vaccination be postponed after the first year as in infancy the immune response may not be satisfactory owing to the presence of circulating maternal antibody. Vaccination should not be done within four weeks of other immunising procedures and should not be done in the pregnant woman. Other contraindications include the presence of intercurrent infection, chronic disease, malignant disease, immunoglobulin deficiencies, patients on steroid therapy or the cytotoxic and immunosuppressive drugs or radiation therapy.

Roseola infantum (Fig. 21.1)

This virus disease affects infants of 6 to 24 months of age, and is often confused with rubella. The patient may be quite ill with a pyrexia of about 39·4°C (103°F), irritability and anorexia. The pyrexia usually lasts about three to five days and as the temperature falls the typical

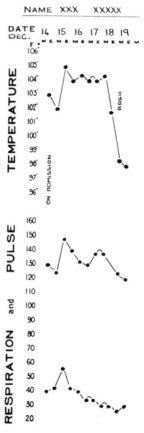

Fig. 21.1 Temperature chart of a case of roseola infantum. Note that the rash appears when the temperature has dropped to normal and the patient has improved.

pink macular 'rose' rash appears on the trunk and limbs; the cervical glands may also be enlarged. The prognosis is good and there is no specific therapy.

Measles (morbilli)

This is a very common acute disease which is extremely infectious. It may affect the infant over the age of 6 months but has its commonest incidence in the older child. The disease is due to a virus and the incubation period is from 7 to 21 days. Clinically the disease may have a prodromal period with pyrexia, irritability and cough. Koplik's spots are found in this early stage and are diagnostic of measles; these spots are tiny, white lesions on a reddened background found on the mucosal surface of the cheek, commonly opposite the molar teeth and best seen by natural light. The prodromal stage is followed by the true disease picture with the typical morbilliform blotchy rash starting behind the ears and spreading over the whole body. The eyes become red and inflamed, and an irritating cough is present in all cases. Various complications such as otitis media, laryngitis, bronchopneumonia and encephalitis may occur.

Treatment

Treatment requires isolation, bed rest and good nursing care. Antibiotic and chemotherapy may be useful in preventing the complications due to secondary infection. Measles virus vaccine (both live attenuated and inactivated killed types) have been developed and are available as agents to actively immunise children against this disease. The live attenuated vaccine (Mevilin) is in general use for active immunisation and as with other vaccines should not be given within four weeks of other vaccine administrations. It should not be used in children who have malignant disease, deficiency of immunoglobins, those undergoing corticosteroid or immunosuppressive treatment, during an acute illness or tuberculosis and should usually not be administered in the first year owing to the presence of circulating maternal antibody in the young infant. Preventive measures may be adopted in susceptible contacts (those not actively immunised) to prevent the disease. For this purpose passive immunity lasting about three weeks may be induced in a susceptible measles contact by injecting human immunoglobulin in the first five days of such contact. Delay in using this material to the sixth to ninth day after contact may attenuate an attack of measles.

Chickenpox (varicella)

This is a virus disease of a highly infectious nature with an incubation period of 14 to 21 days. The patient may be pyrexial and develops the typical vesicular eruption over the whole body most marked on the trunk and face. The mouth may also have these lesions. The lesions start as a macule, become papular then vesicular and finally pustular; they then become crusted. Crops of lesions appear at different times, so that all stages are present at the same time. In smallpox the lesions are all at the same stage of development, and the disease is very much more severe than chickenpox. The rare complication of encephalitis might occur in chickenpox. The disease may be extremely severe in patients receiving corticosteroid therapy. There is no specific treatment for the disease except isolation, bed rest and cooling skin lotions to allay irritation. In especially sensitive susceptible contacts passive immunisation may be induced by administering hyperimmune chickenpox immunoglobulin.

Mumps (epidemic parotitis)

This is an acute infectious disease due to the virus *Myxovirus parotidis*. The incubation period is about 14 to 21 days usually being about 17, but may be longer. It produces an enlarged tender swelling of the parotid gland and is often bilateral. Pyrexia is frequently present and the patient may have difficulty in opening his mouth. This disease may on rare occasions be complicated by meningo-encephalitis or pancreatitis or, in the older age-group, by orchitis. There is no specific treatment except bed rest and a light diet. A mumps vaccine (Mumpsvax) is available for active immunisation. Passive immunisation may be induced by human antimumps immunoglobulin.

Scarlet fever

This condition is caused by a β-haemolytic streptococcus of an erythrogenic strain. The portal of entry is usually the throat but it can follow infection elsewhere such as a wound or a burn ('surgical scarlet fever'). The incubation period is very short—from 1 to 7 days, being usually from 2 to 4 days. The onset is usually sudden with a pyrexia, sore throat and vomiting. The tonsils are usually very congested with some swelling and patches of exudate may appear. The palate may occasionally show petechiae. In the early stages the tongue is covered with a whitish exudate through which the enlarged papillae are seen (strawberry tongue). In a few days the appearance of the tongue changes as the whitish exudate separates leaving a reddish surface with the prominent papillae. The lymph nodes draining the tonsillar area at the angles of the mandible become enlarged, palpable and tender. The skin rash usually appears rapidly and is of a pink erythematous type (punctate erythema); the face is not affected but develops a flush with fairly well-marked pallor around the mouth (circumoral pallor). The rash usually fades gradually after the third day. At the end of the first week the skin peels in a similar sequence to the evolution of the original rash. Areas of desquamation appear on the trunk and cervical areas and eventually extend to the hands and feet. The causative streptococcus may be found on culture from swabs taken from the site of infection such as the throat and the blood count shows a leucocytosis. The antistreptolysin titre rises with this infection.

Various complications may occur in scarlet fever and these include local spread to draining lymph glands producing cervical lymphadenitis and also otitis media. Distant complications by sensitisation are acute glomerulonephritis and rheumatic fever.

The treatment requires bed rest and the administration of penicillin to eradicate the causative haemolytic streptococcus.

Diphtheria

This is an extremely serious disease and is caused by the *Corynebacterium diphtheriae* (Klebs-Loeffler bacillus) organism. The incubation period is short and may extend from 2 to 6 days, being usually 2 to 4 days. The disease is spread by direct droplet infection from 'carriers' and from patients with the disease. The organism produces a toxin which may have disastrous effects on a patient. The onset is usually insidious and during the first week general symptoms are seen. The commonest type of infection is faucial diphtheria where a greyish-white membrane appears at the affected site in the throat. The edges of the membrane are usually well demarcated and there is a surrounding narrow area of redness with the other part of the throat appearing normal. The membrane may extend from the tonsils to the uvula and round the palate. It is firmly attached and can only be forcibly removed after which there is local bleeding. The membrane may also occur in the larynx either as a primary infection at this site or a spread from the pharynx. This laryngeal diphtheria produces dangerous obstruction to breathing with marked inspiratory stridor.

The disease may also affect the nose and this nasal diphtheria is usually mild and is associated with a nasal discharge which may become bloodstained and is usually accompanied by excoriation and crusting of the nostrils. These patients may spread the infection to contacts if they are not isolated.

Diphtheria may be accompanied by serious complications and these patients are often severely ill, having a pyrexia, tachycardia and may develop enlargement of the cervical lymph glands. The toxin of diphtheria may cause damage to the heart and central nervous system and these serious complications have been discussed in other sections of this book.

The differential diagnosis of faucial diphtheria is mainly from infectious mononucleosis but other conditions with membrane in the throat are acute tonsillitis and agranulocytosis. The clinical diagnosis requires confirmation by culturing the causative organism from the areas affected, but it is essential that treatment be commenced as soon as possible.

This urgent treatment of diphtheria should be combined with strict isolation of these patients. The therapy of this condition requires that the toxin be neutralised by the adequate early injection of diphtheria antitoxin in sufficient dosage. The antitoxin dosage is similar for all age-groups and in the mild or moderately severe cases 5000 to 30,000 units is administered intramuscularly. In those cases seen later and in severely affected cases higher doses up to 100,000 units are administered. Special care is required in treating patients with an allergic history and a test dose should be used which is usually given subcutaneously; it may be necessary to use a corticosteroid or adrenalin for the urgent treatment of anaphylactic shock and some patients may be affected later by serum sickness. Prolonged bed rest is necessary for these patients. The organism is usually sensitive to penicillin and erythromycin and in some cases to cephaloridine and these antibiotics are used to eradicate the organism but will have no effect on the toxin for which the antitoxin is essential.

In patients with laryngeal diphtheria the urgent relief of the respiratory obstruction is essential and tracheostomy may be necessary. These patients usually require about 20,000 units of antitoxin. Patients with diphtheria must be strictly isolated until they have had at least three consecutive negative nasal and throat swabs taken at intervals of three days.

Prevention of the disease by active immunisation has become widespread among most communities and the aim should be to immunise all infants against this and other diseases. For this purpose diphtheria toxoid is used. Booster injections are necessary and this is discussed in another section. Tetanus toxoid may be combined to produce immunity against both tetanus and diphtheria. Pertussis vaccine may also be combined but this part of the triple antigen injections given to infants may produce reactions. In the older child toxoid-antitoxin floccules (TAF) in three injections is available for immunisation purposes. The Schick test is available to determine those individuals who are susceptible to diphtheria. This test is performed by injecting intradermally 0·2 ml of the toxin into the forearm and the same volume of heated toxin into the other forearm and their reactions at the injection sites are interpreted in relation to susceptibility or immunity. Susceptible diphtheria contacts may be protected with a small dose of antitoxin for a period of about two weeks (passive immunisation).

Whooping cough (pertussis)

This is an infectious disease with an incubation period of about 14 days. The infection is caused by the *Bordetella pertussis* organism of Bordet-Gengou; this small Gram-negative organism can occasionally be grown from the secretions of acute cases using the cough-plate technique, when the patient is allowed to cough on to a special culture medium contained in a dish. Another technique for obtaining the organism from suspected cases is to examine a posterior pharyngeal swab. The disease may affect any age-group and is most dangerous in the first few months of life.

The clinical features are made up of an initial coryzal-like illness with an irritating cough; this phase is followed by the true disease picture which is associated with the typical spasmodic cough occurring in paroxysms and accompanied by the diagnostic 'whoop' followed by the expectoration of thick mucus, and often vomiting. Variable numbers of these coughing attacks occur in different patients, from a few daily to many in the severe cases. The attacks may last for a few weeks and then become less frequent although even in the convalescent stages of the illness the 'whoop' may still remain. In some cases an ulcer develops below the tongue due to its stretching over the lower incisor teeth during an attack. The disease may be confirmed by isolating the organism using the methods already mentioned or by finding a high lymphocyte count in the blood (lymphocytosis). Various complications may occur, such as bronchopneumonia, patchy atelectatic areas in the lungs due to the thick, viscid plugs of mucus (this may eventually lead to bronchiectasis), convulsions, or the reactivation of a tuberculous focus in the lung. Milder attacks may be caused by *Bordetella parapertussis*.

Treatment requires bed rest in the pyrexial stage with good general nursing care especially aimed at relieving the anxiety of the frightening attacks. Specific therapy in the form of antibiotics such as ampicillin, erythromycin or tetracycline may be useful in reducing the numbers of attacks, especially if used early in the disease.

Active immunisation by using pertussis vaccine, in combination with diphtheria and tetanus antigens, is useful in promoting immunity to the disease. A course of three injections is the usual procedure to adopt in the immunisation of infants. Immunisation in general is correlated and discussed in another section.

Malaria

Although this disease is not an infectious condition it will be briefly discussed here.

It may be caused by various different types of parasite (plasmodium), which are transmitted by the bite of the female anopheles mosquito; malaria therefore only occurs in areas where this mosquito abounds. There are four species of plasmodium (*Plasmodium falciparum, P. vivax, P. malariae* and *P. ovale*). A typical pyrexial illness occurs with sweating, enlargement of the spleen and anaemia; this may be followed by recurrent attacks of fever. The diagnosis is confirmed by finding the malarial parasite in the red cells of stained blood smears. The plasmodium parasite goes through various stages of its life-cycle, partly in the mosquito and partly in man. The disease may take on various severe forms such as the cerebral type of malaria, malignant tertian malaria (*Plasmodium falciparum*). The treatment of the acute attack requires the use of the antimalarial drugs such as chloroquine (Nivaquine, Avloclor), amodiaquine (Camoquin) or proguanil (Paludrine); quinine is useful in the treatment of the pernicious forms of malaria such as cerebral malaria where it is administered as quinine dihydrochloride by slow intravenous injection. Other antimalarial measures require preventive community health action against the mosquito and protection of the individual from the bite of mosquitoes and the use of prophylactic antimalarial drugs in malarial areas such as pyrimethamine (Daraprim).

Typhoid fever (enteric fever)

This is an infection due to *Salmonella typhi*. It has a slow onset with a persistent pyrexia and is associated with ulceration of the lymphoid Peyer's patches of the small bowel. The individual is infected by swallowing the organism contained in contaminated water or foods such as milk. Contamination of foods may occur from a 'carrier' of the

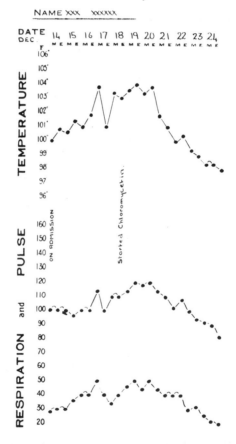

Fig. 21.2 Temperature chart of a patient suffering from typhoid fever treated with chloramphenicol (Chloromycetin). Note that the temperature has fallen to normal after five days of treatment. The drug is continued for a further 10 to 14 days.

organism. In childhood the disease may be milder than in adults but is frequently also severe. In infancy the disease may manifest itself as a gastroenteritis. The infection goes through the various clinical stages of initial rise in temperature ('step-ladder' rise), persistently high temperature with toxaemia and then slow improvement. The stools are often loose and greenish in colour (pea-soup stools). The various complications, though more uncommon in childhood, may also occur; these include bowel haemorrhage or perforation (from the ulcerated Peyer's patches). Typical 'rose-spots' may occur on the skin of the trunk or limbs. The diagnosis may be confirmed by finding *Salmonella typhi* in a blood culture during the first week of the illness, or finding the organism in the stools or urine of the patient. The agglutination reactions (Widal reaction) become positive with a rising titre from the second week onwards. A blood count often shows a leucopenia (lowered white blood cell count).

The treatment of the disease requires careful expert nursing with barrier isolation precautions, a light nourishing diet and observation for complications. Symptomatic treatment is necessary and specific therapy with chloramphenicol (Chloromycetin) orally is required; this drug usually leads to a fall in the temperature in about four to five days, and requires to be given for a further period of 10 to 14 days if a relapse is to be prevented (Fig. 21.2). Ampicillin (Penbritin) may also be effective and also the combination of trimethoprim and sulphamethoxazole (Septrin, Bactrim).

Infection with similar organisms to *Salmonella typhi*, such as *Salmonella paratyphi* A, B or C (*S. paratyphi*, *S. schottmülleri*, *S. hirschfeldii*) may produce a milder but similar clinical picture to that of true typhoid fever. Immunity against these infections may be stimulated by using TAB vaccine inoculations or for typhoid fever only, by using a monovalent typhoid vaccine where the immunity may last up to three years.

Brucellosis (undulant fever, Malta fever)

This disease is caused by *Brucella melitensis* and *Brucella abortus*. The infection may be carried by raw milk or acquired from cattle and goats. It occurs more frequently among farmers and is uncommon in children. The incubation period is from 5 to 30 days. The onset of the illness is usually gradual with headache, fatigue and malaise and this is accompanied by prolonged periods of fluctuating pyrexia. There may be pains in the limbs and the spleen is often palpable. Blood cultures and specific blood agglutination reactions are the usual diagnostic aids. A skin reaction to the intradermal injection of brucellin is usually positive but may not indicate active disease.

Treatment requires the use of the tetracycline antibiotics, with streptomycin added in severe cases.

Leptospirosis

These infections are a group of diseases caused by different types of leptospiral organisms. These organisms include *Leptospira ictero-haemorrhagica* (Weil's disease), *L. canicola* (canicola fever) and *L. autumnalis* (pretibial fever). These leptospiral organisms belong to the spirochaetal group and can be easily cultured. The incubation period is 1 to 2 weeks and infection may occur by exposure to infected animals such as rodents or to their excreta. The symptoms may vary and the onset is usually sudden. The infection may be severe with widespread involvement of liver, kidneys and muscles. The symptomatology includes fever, albuminuria, jaundice, haematuria, anaemia, muscular pain, suffusion of the conjunctivae and skin haemorrhages; neck stiffness may be present and maculopapular skin eruptions may also occur. There may be a temporary remission after which the fever may return with signs of involvement of individual organs. Laboratory tests are available for diagnostic purposes and these include culturing the organism from the blood or cerebrospinal fluid during the first week and later from the urine. After the second week of the illness serological tests will be positive showing a rise in specific antibodies with high titres. Symptomatic treatment is necessary and penicillin should be administered, starting treatment if possible during the first three days of the illness. However, penicillin or other antibiotics may not be very effective.

Congenital syphilis

Infants contract congenital syphilis *in utero*, via the placenta, the spirochaete *Treponema pallidum* being the causative organism. If the infection occurs very early in pregnancy an abortion may follow; if the infection occurs later, the infant may be born either with evidence of the disease or apparently healthy and only develop signs of the disease a few weeks after birth. The clinical features of the condition differ in the young infant from those in the older child.

In the young infant, the child may be small, premature and puny or appear to be fairly healthy at birth. The most important manifestations of the disease in the young infant in the first few months of life are the following:

1. Skin lesions (Fig. 21.3) which are usually of a moist desquamative type affecting mainly the palms of the hands, the soles of the feet and the buttocks. (The creases of the buttocks are affected in contrast to a napkin rash, which affects the prominences of the buttocks in contact with the napkin.) These wet, desquamative lesions before treatment are highly infectious; any person attending to these lesions must take care to protect themselves from infection. The corners of

the mouth become cracked, and later form the typical fissured rhagades.

2. The nose develops 'snuffles' with evidence of a bloodstained nasal discharge. This condition may progress, if untreated, to the saddle-shaped nose of the older congenital syphilitic patient.

3. Laryngitis may develop.

4. Fatal pneumonia alba occurs on rare occasions.

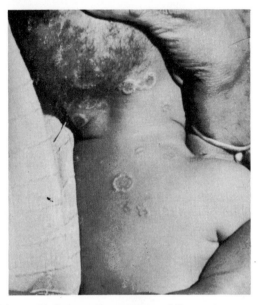

Fig. 21.3 Serpiginous skin lesions of congenital syphilis.

5. Bony lesions frequently occur; these affect the long bones with evidence of periostitis, osteochondritis with bone destruction and epiphysitis. This may be manifested clinically by pain in the affected part and refusal to move that limb (pseudoparalysis). X-ray examination is necessary to indicate the precise changes in the long bones (Figs 21.4 and 21.5).

6. Jaundice may occasionally be present associated with a pericellular cirrhosis of the liver; in addition, the spleen is often enlarged.

7. Anaemia may be present, giving the infant a café-au-lait complexion.

8. Meningitis may rarely occur in early congenital syphilis; this may be associated with convulsions and the diagnosis is confirmed by examination of the cerebrospinal fluid.

9. The blood serology (Wassermann or Kahn reactions) may only become positive about three months after birth, but the mother's Wassermann reaction is always positive. A more accurate blood test for this disease is the *Treponema pallidum* immobilisation test (TPI).

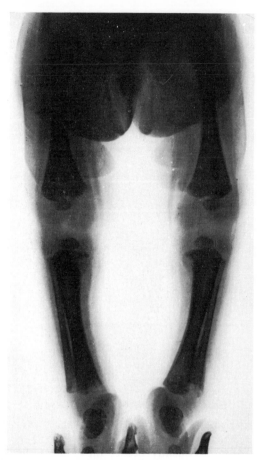

Fig. 21.4 X-ray of the lower limbs of a young infant with congenital syphilis showing generalised periostitis (raising of the periosteum of both femurs, tibiae and fibulae). (*By courtesy from Kessel: 'South African Medical Journal'*.)

In the older child over about 5 years, the patient with congenital syphilis develops different clinical features. These include Hutchinson's triad of symptoms of interstitial keratitis, deafness and the notched peg-shaped permanent central incisor teeth (Hutchinson's teeth). Other manifestations include bilateral painless effusion into the knee joints (Clutton's joints), periosteal thickening of the tibial bones (sabre tibiae) and a perforated palate.

Fortunately this disease has become very uncommon due to the efficient community health and antenatal services which detect and adequately treat pregnant syphilitic women; with efficient treatment in pregnancy these women give birth to normal, non-infected children.

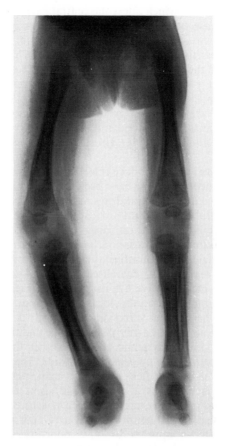

Fig. 21.5 Radiograph of the lower limbs showing the signs of congenital syphilis in a young infant. Note the destruction of bone of the upper medial aspects of both tibiae (Wimberger's sign) and lower ends of tibiae and fibulae and periostitis.

The treatment of the disease in infants and children requires adequate use of penicillin with appropriate follow-up of the clinical signs and serology of these patients.

Virus infections

Virus infections are very common and rapid strides have been made in the study of these diseases (virology). The viruses include the group which affect mainly the skin and mucous membranes which are called dermotropic; typical examples of this type of infection include measles, smallpox and vaccinia (cowpox). Another important group are the neurotropic viruses which affect the central nervous system and include those that cause paralytic poliomyelitis, rabies and encephalitis. The viscerotropic viruses are the causative agents in yellow fever, dengue and virus hepatitis. Another important group of viruses in infancy and childhood are the respiratory types and these include those that cause influenza and psittacosis (parrot fever); the respiratory group also include the adenoviruses and the respiratory syncytial virus. The enteroviruses are a further group of importance to man and have pathogenic effects in childhood and these include the Coxsackie viruses, poliomyelitis and the ECHO viruses (enteric cytopathogenic human 'orphan').

All these viruses can produce infection and disease in childhood and the more important of these have been discussed elsewhere in this book. The development of antiviral drugs has been difficult and this is related to the intracellular life and multiplication of viruses which are protected by the host cell. The antiviral drugs include methisazone which is a thiosemicarbazone preparation. It is active as a prophylactic agent in smallpox contacts but is inactive as treatment for smallpox, but may be useful in the treatment of generalised vaccinia. Another antiviral drug is idoxuridine which is active against certain viruses such as the herpes-virus and is mainly used by local application, for example, in the treatment of herpesvirus infection of the eye; it may also be used in severe infections such as herpesvirus encephalitis and then is given intravenously for its systemic effect. Another drug having a similar action to idoxuridine is cytosine arabinoside. These antiviral drugs are limited in their use by their toxicity to man. Another antiviral drug, amantadine, is useful as a prophylactic agent for influenza virus A infection but is ineffective against influenza virus B. It is possible that its widespread use for influenzal prophylaxis may give rise to resistant viruses. Interferon appears to have poor therapeutic action when infection has started with the influenza virus.

Immunisation with virus vaccines are very effective.

Immunisation

In discussing the measures available to increase the resistance of an individual to infection it is necessary to appreciate immunity responses. This may best be illustrated by the following table:

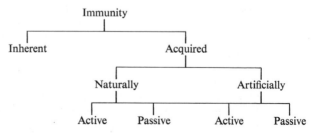

Inherent immunity may be of importance in such conditions as tuberculosis. Naturally acquired passive immunity is seen particularly in the first few months after birth and is acquired by the infant from the mother *in utero* via the placenta. It is well known that the young infant is usually immune to such infections as measles, diphtheria, chickenpox and certain other infections for a period after birth, usually about three to six months; it is of importance to remember that this does not apply to whooping cough and that the newborn infant is susceptible to this dangerous infection at a most vulnerable age.

Naturally acquired active immunity follows certain infections. In the case of some systemic viral infections such as measles, chickenpox and others good life-long immunity usually follows. Variable immunity may follow other types of infection such as poliomyelitis or influenza and this is best explained by the infecting organism being of different types (e.g. polioviruses type I, II or III) where the immunity response is type-specific. In certain other viral infections such as psittacosis there may be no immune response.

Artificially administered passive immunisation is practised in certain problems. Diphtheria antitoxin may be given to susceptible contacts in a dosage of 500 to 2000 units to provide passive immunity lasting about two weeks. Passive immunity against tetanus infection may be provided by the administration of tetanus antitoxin in human tetanus immuno-globulin (Humotet) to injured patients who have not been actively immunised against this dangerous and frequently fatal infection. As antibodies are concentrated in the γ-globulin (gammaglobulin) fraction of the serum proteins it is now common practice to administer by intramuscular injection this product of human origin with the object of providing immune bodies against certain infections. This is available for use in the prevention or attenuation of measles; it is necessary for this human immunoglobulin to be administered within the first five days of measles contact to prevent the attack, and for attenuation a smaller dose may be given from the sixth to the ninth day of contact. Human immunoglobulin may also be useful in the prevention of infective hepatitis in susceptible contacts and also in certain other viral infections such as rubella.

Active artificially acquired immunity is induced by the administration of suitable antigens. This is a most important field in preventive medicine especially in the young child. The efficacy of active immunisa-tion against diphtheria is well exemplified by the statistics of mortality from this disease in England and Wales which dropped from a figure of 2466 in 1940 to 9 in 1954. The agents available for active immunisation against diphtheria are formol toxoid (FT) and adsorbed diphtheria vaccine (BP) on aluminium. It had been recognised in the past that the mineral carrier aluminium was probably the reason for paralytic poliomyelitis developing in the inoculated limb in a child incubating this disease; however, with the falling incidence of poliomyelitis following immunisation, this problem has become of less importance. Refined formol toxoid has been shown to be less efficacious as an immunising agent; the alum preparations are good agents to use and the combined antigens (diphtheria, pertussis, tetanus) act extremely well. FT is useful for the immunisation of the older child.

Pertussis (whooping cough) immunisation is necessary in the young infant because of the danger of this infection in early life but this vaccine can produce reactions and if such a reaction affects the central nervous system (e.g. convulsions) it should not be repeated; furthermore, pertussis immunisation should not be given to the child over 2 years of age. Tetanus toxoid is given for active immunisation and it is an essential in proper preventive medical practice. Efficient immunity responses are obtained by using combined antigenic substances.

Active immunisation against poliomyelitis is widely used. The Sabin type of attenuated live trivalent poliomyelitis virus vaccine is generally available for active immunisation and has met with great success; it is administered by mouth. The Salk type of formolised killed virus vaccine is administered by intramuscular injection from the age of 6 months in a dose of 1 ml followed in a month by the same dose and repeated six to seven months later; a fourth injection is necessary after some years. This has been replaced by the orally administered Sabin-type vaccine, which is administered in three doses at intervals of about six to eight weeks in the first year of life for the first two doses, with the third dose about six months later and a reinforcing dose at school entry.

Vaccination against smallpox was first performed by Edward Jenner in Gloucestershire in 1796. The virus of cowpox is used for this purpose (calf lymph). The infant should be immunised in the first few years of life. Since 1948 vaccination has not been compulsory in the United Kingdom and, furthermore, routine vaccination is not recommended except for selected groups such as the armed forces, health workers and travellers to endemic areas. Vaccination is performed by the minimal trauma technique of a single linear scratch of 3 to 5 mm ($\frac{1}{8}$ to $\frac{1}{4}$ inch) in length or the multiple puncture method of 6 to 20 punctures through a drop of lymph, on the previously cleansed skin. If the vaccination is successful the lesion proceeds through the following stages: a papule on the fourth day, a vesicle on the fifth followed by umbilication on the sixth day; the lesion becomes turbid on the eighth day and forms a pustule with regional adenitis on the tenth day. Crusting of the lesion then develops on the eleventh to the fourteenth day and this separates after approximately 21 days leaving the typical vaccination scar. Vaccination is usually performed over the left deltoid region. Revaccination is necessary every three to seven years in order to maintain proper immunity. Vaccination against smallpox can be associated with certain extremely rare complications; these include generalised vaccinia (Fig. 21.6), localised vaccinia by direct contact from the site of the original vaccination, sepsis from secondary infection and post-vaccinial encephalitis, which, although very rare, is more likely to follow primary vaccination of an older person. Infantile eczema is a contraindication to vaccination as this may precipitate the generalised vaccinial reaction of the Kaposi's varicelliform type (a similar disease may follow herpesvirus infection of an eczematous infant). Vaccination should also not be performed in the presence of a febrile illness, in a child with a septic skin lesion or in a child on corticosteroid therapy.

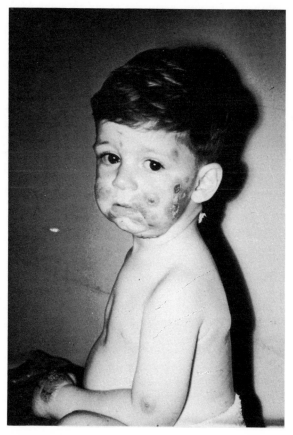

Fig. 21.6 Generalised vaccinia occurring as a complication of vaccination.

With the isolation of the measles virus an attenuated live vaccine and an inactivated (killed) vaccine is available for active immunisation against measles as mentioned elsewhere in this book; the attenuated live vaccine (Melvilin-L) is being extensively used. As also mentioned elsewhere, with the isolation of the rubella virus a live attenuated rubella virus vaccine (Almevax, Cendevax) is available to secure active immunisation against this important cause of congenital abnormalities. In the presence of a typhoid epidemic it may be necessary to actively immunise against this disease by the injection of monovalent typhoid vaccine or TAB vaccine; this provides immunity for approximately three years.

Protective vaccines against rabies, cholera, yellow fever, influenza and plague have been in use for a number of years.

A suitable scheme of immunisation requires three doses of triple antigen (diphtheria, tetanus, pertussis) at six to eight week intervals near the sixth month for the first two injections followed by the third about six months later, with a booster dose at school entry of diphtheria and tetanus only. Three doses of oral poliovirus vaccine are administered in the second six months at six to eight week intervals for the first two followed by the third dose six months later with an additional dose at school entry. Smallpox vaccination is done during the first two years but is not recommended as a routine procedure in the United Kingdom. In the vaccinated individual, revaccination is necessary at suitable intervals. Measles vaccination can be done after the first year and rubella vaccination in females during childhood. BCG vaccine may be administered at any suitable time, depending on circumstances.

22. Common Poisonings in Childhood

Many children are admitted to hospital suffering from the poisonous effects of swallowing many different substances. They accidentally swallow pills and tablets or other materials which are negligently within their reach in many homes. It is important to stress that these cases are always preventable, and the dangers of these happenings should be regularly brought to the public attention who should be educated against these hazards to child life. A useful preventive measure would be to introduce containers which are difficult for children to open and also to make medicinal tablets less attractive to children. Many pills such as iron and others are brightly coloured and attract the attention of young children who may then swallow them with harmful and often tragic results. It is also important to educate the public to keep toxic substances out of the reach of children. All cases of poisoning should be admitted to a hospital for treatment and a period of observation. In many cases gastric lavage is necessary although in the conscious child an emetic such as syrup ipecacuanha may be useful as an alternative. Gastric lavage is not recommended and should not be done for the treatment of poisoning by corrosive and caustic substances and for kerosene poisoning. Poisons information centres have been established in the United Kingdom to provide information in relation to these problems. These centres include that at Guy's Hospital, London (telephone 01-407 7600), The Royal Infirmary, Cardiff (telephone 0222 33101), The Royal Infirmary, Edinburgh (telephone 031-229 2477) and the Royal Victoria Hospital, Belfast (telephone 0232 30503).

Kerosene poisoning (paraffin)

This is a commonly ingested substance and has a tendency to produce a pneumonitis which may only be confirmed by radiological examination of the chest. Gastric lavage should not be performed as experience has proved that those cases not submitted to this procedure do as well as the others. The children with this condition should be carefully nursed and may require an oxygen tent; prophylactic penicillin therapy is useful. The prognosis for these cases is usually very good and very few fatalities occur. If pneumonitis is present X-ray examination is necessary to monitor the improvement.

Barbiturate poisoning

Phenobarbitone is a common barbiturate and often accidentally swallowed as it is a drug found in many homes. The clinical picture of poisoning with phenobarbitone is similar to that produced by any barbiturate. The principal effect is sedation and where large amounts are swallowed a comatose condition is produced, with marked depression of respiratory function. It is possible to accurately estimate the blood barbiturate levels. Gastric lavage is essential as soon as possible. Careful nursing is required and oxygen therapy may be useful; in the comatose patient it is essential to maintain a clear airway. Intravenous infusion to induce diuresis may be very useful as a therapeutic measure. A stimulant drug, bemegride, has been administered intravenously in the treatment of barbiturate poisoning but has been disappointing in its effect in children. In severe cases with marked respiratory depression intermittent positive pressure respiration (IPPR) is essential and may be life-saving. Prophylactic penicillin should be given. Another useful therapeutic procedure in barbiturate poisoning is dialysis.

Salicylism (aspirin poisoning)

Any form of salicylate if ingested in excessive amounts can give rise to salicylism. It most frequently follows the ingestion of aspirin, but the same clinical picture follows the accidental ingestion of such substances as methyl salicylate linament (oil of wintergreen), which contains a large amount of salicylate. Aspirin poisoning may be discussed under three headings:

1. Idiosyncrasy to aspirin may produce different symptoms related to the sensitivity of the drug, and not the clinical picture of salicylism. The various manifestations such as purpura or even angioneurotic oedema may occur and these may even follow minimal dosage of the drug.
2. Accidental ingestion of aspirin tablets by a child is a very common happening. In these cases gastric lavage should be performed as soon as possible using a solution of sodium bicarbonate. There may be a latent period of some hours before the signs of salicylism manifest themselves; if this should occur urgent treatment must be instituted.
3. Therapeutic aspirin poisoning. This type of intoxication most frequently affects the infant under the age of 1 year. These infants usually have some illness such as an upper respiratory tract infection, diarrhoea or other febrile condition for which they are given aspirin, often by the parents. These infants who develop clinical signs of salicylism may also have some sensitivity to the drug.

Clinical features

The clinical signs of salicylism may produce evidence of severe illness and marked hyperventilation. The child often appears shocked and has a pale, greyish appearance; in these circumstances urgent therapy is essential. Haemorrhagic manifestations and convulsions may occur. The diagnosis may be confirmed by the history of having taken aspirin, by the presence of salicylate in the urine (using the Phenistix test) and by estimating the salicylate blood level if laboratory facilities are available. The severity of the illness may be assessed by other laboratory investigations such as the blood gases and the electrolyte levels. Severe salicylism is an extremely dangerous condition with high mortality.

Treatment

As mentioned previously, in cases of accidental ingestion of the drug, gastric lavage with a solution of sodium bicarbonate is essential. In therapeutic cases, however, there is no need to perform a gastric lavage as the ingestion of the aspirin will have gone on for some time in small doses. Severe cases require intravenous therapy and useful fluids to infuse include one-fifth normal saline with 4·3 per cent glucose with the addition of sodium bicarbonate to counteract the acidosis if necessary; the amounts should be carefully controlled and the requirement monitored in relation to the blood gases and electrolyte investigations. Salicylate has a tendency ro reduce the prothrombin content of the blood which may induce bleeding and vitamin K_1 should be administered to counteract this tendency. Penicillin should be used and oxygen therapy may be necessary. Convulsions should be controlled. In desperately ill cases an exchange transfusion may be life saving, and also peritoneal dialysis or haemodialysis might also be used to treat extremely ill patients with this form of poisoning.

Organophosphate insecticide poisoning

This group includes the highly toxic substance parathion, which, if accidentally swallowed, can produce respiratory failure. It has an effect in reducing the cholinesterase and the treatment requires the use of atropine; artificial respiration may be necessary. Gastric lavage is essential. This substance may also be absorbed from the skin or inhaled with severe toxic effects. Another antidote, praldoxime methane sulphomate, has also been recommended to be given intravenously in the treatment of parathion poisoning (25 mg per kg bodyweight intravenously in a 10 per cent solution).

Chlorinated hydrocarbon insecticide poisoning

These substances include DDT, benzene hexachloride (BHC), dieldrin and lindane and are commonly found in many households. When they are accidentally swallowed they produce stimulation of the central nervous system with restlessness and convulsions, followed later by depression with collapse, cyanosis and respiratory failure. Other symptoms may include nausea and vomiting. Gastric lavage is necessary in these cases and treatment is symptomatic.

Phosphorus poisoning

This substance may be present in certain rat poisons and also in matches. It gives rise to oesophageal pain with nausea, vomiting and diarrhoea. Liver toxicity may be produced with hepatic tenderness, jaundice and hepatic failure. Gastric lavage is necessary and the treatment is symptomatic.

Morphine poisoning

Any of the opium derivatives such as morphine and codeine, if swallowed in large doses, may have severe effects. Depression of respiratory function can be produced and the depth of respiration may become shallow and the rate extremely slow. This poor respiratory function may induce cyanosis and this may be followed by circulatory collapse and respiratory failure. Depression of the central nervous system with coma is often present and the pupils contract to pinpoint size. Certain cough mixtures may contain these opiate substances and in overdosage may produce similar effects.

In cases of accidental ingestion gastric lavage is necessary using a dilute solution of potassium permanganate. Oxygen administration and intermittent positive pressure respiration may be necessary. The specific antagonist nalorphine (lethidrone) should be administered by intramuscular injection and is effective in the treatment of this condition (0·2 mg per kg bodyweight). An appropriate laboratory test makes use of spectrophotometry of the blood or urine.

Caustic soda poisoning

This potentially corrosive substance may be accidentally swallowed by children. Caustic soda is found in many households and there is often insufficient care taken in its control. If it is swallowed, there is a destructive, corrosive effect on the mouth, throat, pharynx and stomach. Initially there may be a severe degree of shock but later the oesophageal effect takes precedence. If the patient survives the initial period, the corrosive effect on the oesophagus leads to contraction and stricture formation with difficulty in swallowing. As with all corrosive poisonings, gastric lavage must not be performed. An initial antidote should be given in the form of a weak acid such as vinegar. The ensuing shock must be treated and an appropriate antibiotic used to prevent infection of the affected part. Early consultation with an oesophagoscopist should be arranged so that oesophageal dilatations may be started soon if the oesophagus is severely affected. Treatment with corticosteroids is also used in an attempt to inhibit scar formation of the oesophagus at the affected site.

Belladonna poisoning (atropine)

The berries of deadly nightshade contain an atropine-like substance and accidental ingestion of these may give rise to atropine or belladonna poisoning. The symptoms are usually very dramatic and include an extreme form of hyperexcitability often bordering on acute mania. In addition, an erythematous rash occurs and also hyperpyrexia, tachycardia, widely dilated pupils, a dry mouth and abdominal pain with possible retention of urine. The treatment of this condition should include gastric lavage, followed by sedation with a short-acting barbiturate such as quinalbarbitone (Seconal). It is necessary to stress that a long-acting sedative should not be used as this may act sufficiently long to combine its sedation effects with the later depressant effects of the atropine-like poison. Pilocarpine is a specific antidote to atropine but only affects the peripheral effect of the poison, such as the dry mouth and dilated pupils, and has no action on the central effect. Neostigmine is also given by mouth. If depression should occur in atropine poisoning, the patient should be stimulated.

Aniline dye poisoning

These dyes are contained in some marking inks, dyes and solvents and may be absorbed if in contact with the skin. It may affect young infants and the low birth weight infants producing an intense cyanosis due to methaemoglobinaemia, which interferes with proper oxygenation of the individual. The treatment requires the use of methylene blue in a 1 per cent solution administered by slow intravenous injection in a dose of 1 to 2 mg per kg bodyweight. An appropriate laboratory test would be spectroscopy of the blood for the presence of methaemoglobin. Vitamin C is also used and in severe cases exchange transfusion may be necessary.

Iron poisoning

Therapeutic pills containing iron, such as ferrous sulphate, are often brightly coloured and attractive to children and may be swallowed accidentally. The iron may have a corrosive effect on the stomach and duodenal mucosa with the development of shock, haemorrhage and death. Vomiting often occurs and a certain amount may be removed by this happening. The iron may also be absorbed and interfere with cellular metabolism producing convulsions and may also be fatal. Immediate gastric lavage is essential and this should be done using a solution of desferrioxamine (2 g per litre). This substance desferrioxamine (Desferal) is a chelating agent and is useful in the treatment of acute iron poisoning and may be administered orally and also intravenously. Treatment for shock may also be necessary where this happens.

Arsenic poisoning

This substance is a common ingredient of ant poisons and may be accidentally swallowed by children. The symptoms induced by this poisoning include vomiting, diarrhoea and shock and death may follow. Immediate lavage of the stomach is essential and dimercaprol may be used. Fluids must be given and dimercaprol should be administered by intramuscular injection in a dosage of about 2·5 to 3·5 mg per kg bodyweight per dose for six to eight injections at six- to eight-hourly intervals. An appropriate laboratory test includes the analysis of the vomitus or stool for arsenic.

Boric acid poisoning

These cases have been reported more frequently and are due to close apposition to areas of skin, of ointments and powders containing boric acid, and another possible source has been borax glycerine. Intoxication may produce diarrhoea and vomiting and an extensive exfoliative skin condition may develop. Neurological signs such as neck retraction and convulsions may occur. In view of the danger of intoxication, preparations containing boric acid, borax and boracic acid should not be used in infancy. In severe cases peritoneal dialysis may be necessary. An appropriate laboratory test would be the estimation of boron in the blood.

Digitalis poisoning

This may follow the accidental ingestion of a digitalis preparation such as digoxin or may be the result of overdosage. The symptoms include vomiting, headache, malaise and visual signs; drowsiness may also be present and the electrocardiogram may show bradycardia, coupled beats or block. Gastric lavage or induced vomiting is necessary following the accidental ingestion of this substance and the subsequent treatment may require the intravenous infusion of potassium in a slow drip, at the same time taking great care that the plasma potassium level does not rise to dangerously high levels. Procainamide may be helpful to control arrhythmia and in severe cases if congestive cardiac failure is not present a beta-receptor-blocking agent such as propanolol (Inderal) (1 mg per kg bodyweight orally) may be used. Blood levels of digoxin can be determined.

Tricyclic drug poisoning

Tricyclic drugs are commonly used in the treatment of depression and include amitriptyline and imipramine. They may be accidentally swallowed and may have a direct effect on the myocardium. The symptoms include drowsiness, ataxia, tachycardia and coma. It is necessary to induce vomiting or do a gastric lavage although this may need to be postponed if cardiac arrhythmia is present. Lignocaine or procainamide are useful for the cardiac effects. In severe cases oxygen and artificial ventilation are necessary.

Monoamine oxidase inhibitors (MAOI)

These are present in many preparations which are used in the treatment of depression. Their effects may be potentiated by foods which contain tryptamine such as cheese, yeast extracts, Marmite, and some drugs. The potentiating effect may induce severe and dangerous reactions resulting in a severe hypertensive crisis, and the possibility of an intracranial haemorrhage. In the accidental ingestion of these substances gastric lavage is essential and a clear airway must be maintained; intermittent positive pressure respiration may be necessary, and the hypertension should be treated with a suitable hypotensive agent.

Antihistamine drug poisoning

These commonly used antihistamine substances may also be accidentally swallowed. They may produce stimulation of the central nervous system, and in these circumstances the judicious use of a very short-acting barbiturate in appropriate dosage is useful in treatment; if depression is produced, the patient must be stimulated. These cases require immediate gastric lavage in an attempt to remove as much of the drug as possible before its absorption.

Lead poisoning (plumbism)

This condition may occur in childhood and may be due to the swallowing of lead-containing paint from old houses, from cots or the sucking of lead toys. Many years ago a possible cause was the use of lead nipple shields by the lactating mother. Lead poisoning may produce lead encephalopathy with convulsions and subsequent brain damage. The treatment for this condition requires a restriction of fluids and the use of intravenous mannitol in a dose of 2 g per kg bodyweight administered in a 25 per cent solution. Anaemia may be present and the erythrocyte protoporphyrin is raised and the urine has an excess of coproporphyrins; punctate basophilia may be found in the red blood cells. An X-ray of the bone ends may show a typical dense line. Confirmation of the diagnosis may be obtained by estimating the lead level of the blood (the normal level is less than 1.7 μmol per litre). The use of sodium calcium edetate may be useful in the management of lead poisoning as also may be D-penicillamine.

Paraquat poisoning

Paraquat is widely used as a weedkiller. It may be accidentally ingested and if absorbed can cause irreversible changes in the lungs. It may be locally corrosive in the mouth, pharynx and oesophagus and it can also have an effect on the liver and kidney. The estimated fatal dose is 4 mg per kg bodyweight. Urgent gastric lavage is necessary and it may be useful to use a solution of bentonite (BP). This should be followed by forced diuresis in an attempt to rapidly eliminate the absorbed toxic substance from the body. The immunosuppressive drugs and the corticosteroids have been used but with little benefit. The irreversible lung changes have led to lung transplantation in an attempt to salvage these patients.

Naphthalene poisoning

This substance is present in many moth repellants and may be accidentally swallowed. It can cause haemolysis thereby producing haemoglobinuria and is often associated with nausea, vomiting and diarrhoea. The haemolysis may lead to anaemia and convulsions might also occur. Immediate gastric lavage is necessary and general supportive treatment; in very severe cases exchange transfusion may be necessary.

Turpentine poisoning

Turpentine may be accidentally swallowed and can cause severe abdominal pain. It is often associated with vomiting and diarrhoea and respiratory symptoms might also occur. It requires gastric lavage and general supportive treatment.

Carbon monoxide poisoning

This gas poisoning has an effect by producing carboxyhaemoglobin in the blood and thereby interfering with oxygen carriage causing anoxia. It is associated with headache, dizziness, weakness and unconsciousness. A typical cherry-red colour of the lips and fingers develops. The presence of carboxyhaemoglobin in the blood may be confirmed by spectroscopic examination. These patients require urgent respiratory support and oxygenation and for this purpose the use of hyperbaric oxygen may be extremely useful.

Carbon tetrachloride poisoning

This substance is commonly found in cleaning liquids and if accidentally swallowed may produce severe symptoms of abdominal pain, vomiting, diarrhoea, jaundice and anuria. Appropriate laboratory investigations should include liver function tests. The treatment requires general and supportive measures including the use of calcium gluconate solutions given slowly intravenously, and in severe cases haemodialysis.

23. Common Paediatric Procedures

In the practice of paediatrics there are many procedures which are essential and necessary for the investigation and management of many diseases. These include the techniques of taking blood for investigations, the collection of urine and many other procedures which will be briefly discussed. It is necessary that children should be adequately sedated for many of these procedures.

Blood may be obtained from different veins; in the older child it may be obtained by puncture of the cubital vein at the elbow. For all procedures performed on infants and children it is essential that proper restraint be used and this fact cannot be sufficiently stressed. In infants difficulty may be experienced in obtaining blood at the elbow, and in these circumstances the external or the internal jugular vein or the femoral vein in the inguinal region may be used. Internal jugular vein puncture is a blind procedure but is a satisfactory method of obtaining blood in efficient and trained hands. The operator, however, must be aware of its dangers which are related to the proximity of various important structures in the neck.

For the intravenous infusion of fluids, blood or plasma the appropriate vein may be punctured by a 'push-in' with a suitable needle. The veins at the elbow may be efficiently used in the older child, but in the infant the veins on the dorsum of the hand should be used; if these fail, a scalp vein puncture may be successful, and in these cases a sharp, short, short-bevel needle should be used. If these techniques fail a 'cut-down' on a vein must be performed and this surgical exposure is usually done on the saphenous vein at the ankle and a plastic cannula should be inserted.

For the occasional use of subcutaneous infusion of fluids a needle should be inserted into the tissues of the thighs or the interscapular region or the flanks. Half-strength saline solutions may be given by this technique and it is advantageous to use hyaluronidase to hasten the absorption of the fluids.

The procedure of exchange transfusion is used in the treatment of haemolytic disease of the newborn or hyperbilirubinaemia. This is usually efficiently performed via the umbilical vein soon after birth. In cases of difficulty the femoral vein in the inguinal region may be used after its surgical exposure.

The procedure of lumbar puncture is necessary to obtain cerebrospinal fluid, and this is performed between the third and fourth lumbar vertebrae or one space lower. It is essential that the patient should be held quite still, either lying on the side or sitting up. A subdural haematoma or effusion may be diagnosed and treated by the procedure of subdural tapping. These conditions may occur in infants after trauma (birth trauma or subsequently) or may follow a pyogenic meningitis such as the *Haemophilus influenzae* type. This procedure can only be performed on infants where the anterior fontanelle is still patent. The needling of the subdural space is performed with absolutely sterile precautions through the suture line at the lateral angle of the anterior fontanelle, penetrating the dural membrane at a depth of about 3 mm.

Gastric lavage may be necessary as a diagnostic or therapeutic procedure; in these cases the appropriate-size tube should be passed through the mouth. A similar procedure is necessary in oesophageal tube feeding. In the past it was necessary to intubate the duodenum in order to obtain fluid to test for the presence of the exocrine secretions of the pancreas (pancreatic enzymes) in doubtful cases of cystic fibrosis but at the present time the iontophoretic collection of sweat for salt content estimation has replaced the need for duodenal intubation in the diagnosis of this disease. The peroral suction duodenojejunal biopsy investigation was developed as a technique for the investigation of malabsorption disorders by Margot Shiner and this investigation requires the use of the Crosby-Kugler capsule or its modification. Various endoscopic investigations are being used in children and these investigations require the use of various types of fibroscope, such as the gastrointestinal type or the colonofibroscope to do colonoscopy (Figs. 23.1 and 23.2).

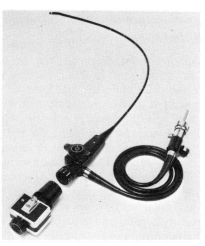

Fig. 23.1 Forward viewing paediatric gastroduodenofibrescope. (*By courtesy of KeyMed Specialised Medical Equipment Ltd.*)

The collection of urine in infants may be difficult. Patience may be rewarded by intercepting a naturally voided specimen. A cottonwool swab may be applied in the female infant to collect urine and then squeezed out to provide sufficient non-sterile urine for some clinical tests; a special receptacle for the collection of urine from female children is available. In male infants a sterile test-tube can be used to collect a specimen. A special disposable plastic urine collector for male and female infants and children is now available for the efficient collection of urine for investigation. Bladder puncture urine may be obtained by the suprapubic puncture of the bladder when a specimen of urine can be obtained under sterile conditions.

Neurological diagnosis includes the technique of computerised axial tomography using the EMI brain scanner. This method is extremely useful to detect brain lesions such as tumour, hydrocephaly, subdural effusion and other diseases.

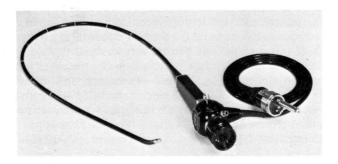

Fig. 23.2 Side viewing paediatric gastrofibrescope. (*By courtesy of Keymed Specialised Medical Equipment Ltd.*)

Bone marrow specimens for diagnosis may be obtained by bone marrow puncture at various sites. In small infants a suitable site is the tibial bone and in the older child the iliac crest or vertebral spinous process may be punctured. In the near adolescent the sternum may be used in the same way as in the adult. A marrow trephine may also be performed using a bone-marrow trephine needle and trocar.

Various other procedures are carried out in infancy and childhood similar to those done on adults. These procedures include abdominal, thoracic or pericardial paracentesis and other procedures, the principles and precautions for which are similar to their performance on adult patients. Hepatic and renal needle biopsy examination are a necessary investigation in certain hepatic and renal diseases, and these may be carried out where proper facilities for such investigations are available.

24. A Short Account of Antimicrobial Agents

Penicillin

Penicillin is probably the best antibiotic agent in use. Its main disadvantage is the possible allergic effect on sensitive individuals. The original penicillin was obtained from the mould *Penicillium notatum*. Of the original four types of penicillin which were known, benzyl-penicillin (penicillin G) is the most active. It is administered usually by intramuscular injection, but has been used orally in buffered form as benzathine penicillin. It is also given by intravenous infusion, by aerosol methods, injection into closed spaces (very rarely at the present time into the intrathecal space—then only in small amounts of about 10,000 units of pure crystalline penicillin G well diluted) and by topical application (e.g. on the skin or in the eye). Various long-acting penicillin preparations are available allowing for less frequent administration to the patient.

A group of British research workers have isolated the basic nucleus—6-aminopenicillanic acid; from this nucleus different types of penicillins have been synthesised. Some of these are acid-stable and are not destroyed by the gastric juices of the stomach; they can therefore be administered by mouth. Some appear also to be active against penicillin-resistant staphylococci. The first to be developed was phenoxyethyl-penicillin, or phenethicillin (Broxil, Bendralan). This is acid-stable and is administered by mouth. The second to be developed was dimethoxy-phenylpenicillin, or methicillin (Celbenin, Staphcillin). This substance has the ability to be active and stable in the presence of penicillinase and is therefore of great value in the treatment of resistant staphylococcal infections. It is not acid-stable and must therefore be administered by intramuscular injection. The third therapeutically useful substance derived from the penicillin nucleus was ampicillin (Penbritin). This is acid-stable and is used orally; this preparation has a wider range of activity than the original penicillin G, being active against both Gram-positive and Gram-negative organisms. Amoxycillin (Amoxil) is similar to ampicillin but needs smaller dosage. Other synthetic penicillins in general use are cloxacillin (Orbenin), flucloxacillin (Floxapen) and oxacillin (Prostaphlin); these are also resistant to penicillinase and are acid-stable, allowing for oral administration. Another penicillin

257

derivative is carbenicillin (Pyopen) for injection use which is active against *Pseudomonas pyocyanea* and Proteus organisms. A derivative of carbenicillin known as carfecillin (Uticillin) is available for certain urinary infections but resistance may develop. Other related preparations such as ticarcillin, talampicillin and hetacillin have also been available for clinical use. Before these synthetic penicillins were developed, phenoxymethylpenicillin (penicillin V) became available; this is acid-stable and is of great use as an orally administered penicillin. Penicillin is bactericidal in its action as is streptomycin, kanamycin, bacitracin and polymyxin, having a sterilising effect in contrast to other antibiotics in use which have a bacteriostatic effect and suppress multiplication of bacteria.

Side-effects. These have been few although more reports have appeared recording severe, grave and sometimes fatal reactions to penicillin; the usual type of reaction is an allergic one affecting the skin. These usually respond well to the antihistamine drugs. Sensitivity reactions may also follow the topical application of the antibiotic to the skin or other parts. Penicillinase (Neutrapen) is available as a therapeutic agent in the treatment of sensitivity reactions to penicillin. Sensitive persons handling the drug are also liable to develop allergic effects.

Chloramphenicol (Chloromycetin)

This antibiotic was first isolated in 1947 from a species of Streptomyces (*Streptomyces venezuelae*) and is now chemically synthesised. It has a broad antibacterial action but its main use is in typhoid fever. In addition, it is also used in cases of influenzal meningitis and other infections resistant to other agents. The drug has a bacteriostatic action. The restricted use for this antibiotic is stressed on account of the possible severe toxic depressive effect on the bone marrow. This very rare happening of bone marrow depression may produce a fatal aplastic anaemia; this effect, although so rare, should restrict the use of this drug to specific conditions. Premature and newborn infants may be severely affected by this drug; a symptom complex known as the grey syndrome has been reported in this age-group where chloramphenicol has been used in the normal therapeutic dosage as recommended for older patients. In this syndrome the infants show a clinical picture of vomiting, refusal of feeds, abdominal distension, respiratory distress and an ashen-grey colour. It is often fatal within a relatively short period. It is essential therefore that chloramphenicol should only be used in the newborn infant, both premature and full-term, where specially indicated and then in low dosage only.

Streptomycin

This antibiotic was discovered in 1944 by Waksman and isolated from *Streptomyces griseus*. It is a bacteriostatic drug in low concentration and also bactericidal. It has a synergistic effect with penicillin on certain organisms (synergism between drugs implies the ability of two drugs to increase their bactericidal effect more than the single drug alone). Streptomycin is not absorbed from the bowel or aerosol inhalation and must therefore be administered for systemic effect by intramuscular injection. It should never be given intravenously because of possible renal damage. It is excreted by the kidneys and in renal disease can build up to toxic levels. It does not normally cross the blood–cerebrospinal fluid barrier and only reaches the cerebrospinal fluid in the presence of meningeal inflammation. It should be used with care in newborn and premature infants. Its main use is in the treatment of tuberculosis but it is also used in certain infections due to Gram-negative organisms. When given by intramuscular injection it is usually administered in a dose of 20 to 40 mg per kg bodyweight per 24 hours; this dosage may be increased in severe cases such as tuberculous meningitis or miliary tuberculosis. The maximum dose in a child should never exceed 1 g per 24 hours. In a few cases of tuberculous meningitis it is still administered by intrathecal injection but there is a very small need for this at the present time; when given intrathecally, the dosage in children is usually 1 mg per kg bodyweight per day. It is also used orally for its local effect on certain infections of the bowel and in these cases there is little systemic absorption from the intestinal tract. Streptomycin is combined with tetracycline in the treatment of brucellosis and with isoniazid (INAH) in the treatment of tuberculosis. Unfortunately streptomycin has certain toxic effects, the main one being on the eighth cranial nerve. Both vestibular function (balance) and hearing may be affected. It appears that the vestibular (balance) effect is proportional to the duration of administration, total amount given and the age of the patient. It is seldom seen where treatment is not given for longer than seven days and usually recovers in children. Hearing effects also require more than a week's treatment. Streptomycin might also have allergic sensitivity effects producing skin rashes, angioneurotic oedema, asthma and eosinophilia (increased eosinophils in the blood); drug fever may also be produced by streptomycin. Bacterial organisms may also develop resistance to this drug.

Kanamycin (Kannasyn, Kantrex)

This antibiotic was isolated from *Streptomyces kanamyceticus* in Japan in 1957. It has a bactericidal effect and appears to be effective against staphylococci, *Salmonella*, *Shigella*, coliform and *Proteus* organisms. It does not appear to be effective against streptococci, pneumococci or anaerobic bacteria. It is poorly absorbed from the bowel. It is also administered by intramuscular injection and is excreted by the kidney. Kanamycin may have toxic effects, the most serious being ototoxic affecting hearing and balance, and nephrotoxic affecting the kidney. Mild eosinophilia and skin rashes might also be produced. By intramuscular injection the dose recommended is usually 15 mg per kg bodyweight in 24 hours in divided doses. This dose must be reduced in patients with kidney dysfunction. In the newborn period the dose must also be lower. The drug may also be used orally for bowel sterilisation and in this regard it may be effective for certain bowel infections. In these cases the recommended dose is 50 mg per kg bodyweight per day in four doses.

Erythromycin (Erythrocin, Ilotycin, Ilosone)

This antibiotic was produced in 1952 and is derived from *Streptomyces erythreus*. It is similar in effect to the antibiotics oleandomycin and spiramycin. It has been modified for better absorption by the production of erythromycin estolate, which is the lauryl sulphate salt of propionyl erythromycin (Ilosone). For intravenous use the lactobionate salt (Erythrocin IV) has been prepared; the ethylsuccinate preparation (Erythrocin IM) has been prepared for intramuscular use. Erythromycin is usually prescribed for oral administration; it has a larger antibacterial range than penicillin as it includes the diphtheria, clostridia, rickettsial and haemophilus organisms. It may have mild side-effects and in large dosage may produce nausea, vomiting and diarrhoea. It has been suggested that prolonged use of the lauryl sulphate salt may produce jaundice by a toxic effect on the liver. Erythromycin is a drug which is useful for the treatment of diphtheria carriers.

Neomycin

This antibiotic was isolated from a species of *Streptomyces*. It is bactericidal to both Gram-positive and Gram-negative organisms. It is poorly absorbed from the bowel and may therefore be used for its local effect in bowel infection and to sterilise the bowel in liver failure or prior to bowel surgery. The usual dose recommended for this purpose is 50 mg per kg bodyweight per day in divided doses for seven days. After prolonged oral use malabsorption symptoms may supervene. It should not be used by intramuscular injection as it is ototoxic and nephrotoxic when used systemically. When given intraperitoneally or intrapleurally it can produce respiratory arrest. It has use as a topical agent for certain skin infections and in ophthalmology.

Paromomycin (Humatin)

This antibiotic, isolated from *Streptomyces*, has a bacteriostatic and a bactericidal effect. It is nephrotoxic when given systemically and should only be used in its oral non-absorbable form. It is effective in intestinal amoebiasis and against certain intestinal infections by bacteria such as *Shigella*, *Salmonella* and pathogenic forms of *Escherichia coli*.

Griseofulvin fine particle (Grisovin)

This antibiotic has been introduced into medical practice for its effect on certain forms of fungal infections of the skin, nails or scalp such as tinea capitis (ringworm). It is very useful and is given by mouth for a period of some weeks.

Amphotericin B (Fungizone)

This antibiotic is derived from a species of *Streptomyces* and is an antifungal agent. It is poorly absorbed from the bowel. It is useful for mycotic (fungal) disease and is administered by intravenous infusion. It is indicated in such diseases as disseminated moniliasis (candidiasis), histoplasmosis, blastomycosis, coccidioidomycosis and cryptococcus meningitis (torulosis). Unfortunately this drug may have severe toxic effects on kidney function, or may produce anaemia, diarrhoea and skin rashes; it should only be used where definitely indicated. It is also available for oral and topical use in local monilial infections.

Nystatin (Nystan, Mycostatin)

This is an antimonilial antibiotic and is poorly absorbed from the intestinal tract. It is available for oral administration in the treatment of thrush, and it is also available for topical use in ointment form for monilial conditions of the skin.

Novobiocin (Albamycin, Cathomycin)

This antibiotic is effective against *Staphylococcus aureus* and also against *Proteus* organisms. Drug resistance tends to develop but it may be useful in penicillin-resistant staphylococcal disease. This antibiotic may play a part in inducing jaundice in the newborn.

Tetracycline

Various forms of this antibiotic are known. In 1948, chlortetracycline (Aureomycin) was isolated from *Streptomyces aureofaciens*; in 1950, oxytetracycline (Terramycin) was isolated from *Streptomyces rimosus*. In 1952, tetracycline (Tetrex, Achromycin) became available for therapeutic use. In 1957, demeclocycline (Ledermycin) was produced and has been available in clinical medicine since 1959. This group of antibiotic has a wide range of antimicrobial activity and has a bacteriostatic effect (suppresses multiplication of bacteria). It has an effect on both Gram-positive and Gram-negative organisms, rickettsial infections, and the larger viruses such as psittacosis and also the *Mycoplasma pneumoniae* (Eaton agent), causing primary atypical pneumonia. It is absorbed from the bowel and excreted by the kidneys. It may have side-effects, such as nausea, vomiting and diarrhoea, with an overgrowth of monilia; on rare occasions a severe diarrhoea may be caused by an overgrowth of a resistant strain of *Staphylococcus aureus* (staphylococcal enterocolitis). The tetracycline group of drugs may also stain the teeth and bones of the very young (Fig. 24.1); a reduction of

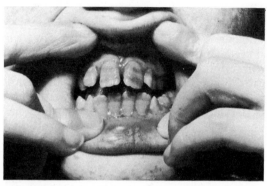

Fig. 24.1 Discoloration and staining of the teeth due to tetracycline administration in early childhood.

bone growth in premature infants has also been recognised. Drug fever and skin rashes may also be produced by this group of antibiotic and it has been suggested that demeclocycline (Ledermycin) may produce photosensitivity of the skin (reaction to sunshine) in certain patients. Certain types of outdated tetracycline can also produce toxic effects.

Gentamicin

This antibiotic belongs to the aminoglycoside group of antimicrobial substances and is bactericidal. It has a wide range of activity against Gram-positive organisms such as *Staphylococcus aureus* and also Gram-negative bacteria such as *Proteus, E. coli, Salmonella, Shigella* and *Pseudomonas*. This antibiotic may be given intramuscularly, intravenously, intrathecally, by aerosol or by topical application. It is almost entirely eliminated from the system by the kidney and serum levels are therefore dependent on renal function. If high blood levels occur toxic effects may follow and these are mainly ototoxic causing deafness and ataxia. It is necessary that blood levels be monitored to keep them between 2 and 10 μg per ml. Gentamicin is an extremely useful antibiotic in appropriate cases.

The cephalosporins

There are various cephalosporins available for clinical use. These include cephaloridine (Ceporin), cephalothin (Keflin) and cephalexin (Ceporex, Keflex). The first two preparations are given by injection and cephalexin is given orally. They have been developed from a basic acid nucleus and they are bactericidal and have a broad spectrum being active against Gram-negative and Gram-positive bacteria such as streptococci, staphylococci and clostridian types. These cephalosporins act at the cell wall and are not cross-allergic with penicillin. They do penetrate into the cerebrospinal fluid and they also cross the placenta. They are useful for patients who are hypersensitive to penicillin. They may produce certain toxic effects such as rashes and eosinophilia. In adults they may be nephrotoxic especially if they are given in large doses with frusemide as a diuretic. It is also reported that a positive Coombs' test may develop and cephaloridine may prolong the prothrombin time.

Lincomycin

This is an antibiotic which is derived from *Streptomyces lincolnensis* and is available as lincomycin hydrochloride (Lincocin, Mycivin) and also as its analogue clindamycin (Dalacin C). These lincomycins are bactericidal and have a broad spectrum against Gram-positive organisms such as streptococci, staphylococci and pneumococci. It is well absorbed from the bowel and is excreted in the urine and bile. Clindamycin can only be given orally and should not be used in early infancy.

Sodium fusidate (Fucidin)

Fusidic acid was extracted from *Fusidium coccineum* and sodium fusidate is an antibiotic which is bactericidal against Gram-positive organisms such as staphylococci, clostridia and the corynebacteria. This antibiotic has no cross-resistance with others and is used in the treatment of staphylococcal infections. It is excreted mainly in the bile and may be given orally or intravenously and also by local topical application. It diffuses very well in the body but not into the urine.

Colomycin (Colistin)

This antibiotic is polymyxin E and was isolated from the *Bacillus colistinus* and is effective against Gram-negative organisms such as *E. coli* and *Pseudomonas* and also *Klebsiella aerogenes*. This antibiotic acts on the cell membrane and is given intramuscularly, intravenously or intrathecally; when given orally it has a local effect on the bowel.

The sulphonamides

There are many sulphonamide preparations available and these chemotherapeutic drugs are useful in medical practice. They were first introduced in 1935 by Domagk, who used the substance prontosil. There are basically three groups of sulphonamides. The first group are rapidly absorbed and rapidly excreted and include sulphadimidine, sulphadiazine, sulphafurazole (Gantrisin) and sulphasomidine (Elkosin). The second group are also rapidly absorbed but more slowly excreted and therefore have a longer action; these include sulphadimethoxine (Madribon) and sulphamethoxypyridazine (Midicel). The third group are the 'non-absorbed' types which include succinylsulphathiazole (Sulfasuxidine), sulphaguanadine and phthalylsulphathiazole (Thalazole); these are poorly absorbed and are used for their local effect in bowel infections such as dysentery. The sulphonamide drugs are bacteriostatic in action and act by competition and interference with its incorporation into folic acid. They have a broad spectrum and affect both Gram-positive and Gram-negative organisms. They should not be used in low birth weight infants or in the newborn or where toxic effects have previously occurred with their use. They are not effective against virus infections, spirochaetes, rickettsial infections or tuberculosis. They are very effective therapeutic agents for meningococcal and nocardial infections, although certain meningococci have become resistant to the sulphonamide drugs in which case penicillin is the drug of choice. They may also be useful in rheumatic fever prophylaxis in patients who are sensitive to penicillin. The sulphonamide drugs are also useful in association with other drugs in such conditions as actinomycosis and pneumococcal meningitis. The sulphonamides are eliminated as metabolic products and are mostly excreted in the urine. They have a low solubility and increased fluid intake is necessary when sulphonamide treatment is given. The sulphonamides do have certain toxic effects which include skin rashes, leucopenia, nausea, purpura, drug fever and haematuria (rarely with anuria). A fairly soluble sulphonamide to use is sulphadimidine (sulphamezathine). A possible toxic effect in the newborn infant, especially with a low birth weight, is to produce a toxic form of jaundice complicated by bilirubin encephalopathy (kernicterus); this type has occurred with the use of sulphafurazole (Gantrisin).

A combination of sulphamethoxazole and trimethoprim in the ratio of 5:1 has a complementary bacteriostatic effect and is available as co-trimoxazole (Septrin, Bactrim). It is rapidly absorbed by the oral route and is mainly secreted in the urine and is effective against both Gram-positive and Gram-negative organisms. It is particularly useful in urinary tract and respiratory tract infections and the organisms against which it is effective include the *Streptococcus, Staphylococcus, Haemophilus, Salmonella, Escherichia* and *Proteus* organisms. There may be toxic effects which include skin rashes, nausea, vomiting and diarrhoea and glossitis. The dose of co-trimoxazole is 1 to 2 mg per kg bodyweight per day of trimethoprim and 5 to 10 mg per kg bodyweight of sulpha-methoxazole.

Another sulphonamide derivative, salicylazosulphapyridine (Salazo-pyrin, Azulfidine, sulphasalazine), is used in the treatment of ulcerative colitis. The benefit from this drug may possibly be due to a local immunosuppressive effect, rather than antibacterial, and is continued for many months after the restoration of normal bowel function in these patients.

An effective drug in the treatment of tuberculosis is rifampicin (Rifadin) which is active at low concentrations against *Mycobacterium tuberculosis* and is used in combination with other antituberculosis drugs. It is administered by mouth and is rapidly absorbed. Rifampicin may produce a reddish discoloration of the urine and lacrimal fluid as a side-effect.

Nitrofurantoin (Furadantin)

This chemical agent is absorbed from the bowel and excreted rapidly by the kidney and has a therapeutic effect on the urinary tract. It is effective against Gram-negative and *Proteus* organisms. The dose is 5 to 7 mg per kg bodyweight per day. Possible side-effects include rashes, gastritis and haemolytic episodes.

Nalidixic acid (Negram)

This preparation is used for urinary infections and is active against *E. coli* and *Proteus* infections. It is given by mouth and excreted in the urine. It may produce side-effects such as nausea, vomiting and skin rashes.

Antiviral drugs

Drugs are becoming available for the prevention and treatment of virus infections. Methisazone (Marboran) is available as a prophylactic agent against smallpox developing in susceptible contacts and as treatment for certain complications of vaccination. Idoxuridine (Kerecid, Dendrid) is a useful drug for the treatment of herpes simplex lesions such as corneal ulcers; other drugs such as amantadine are being developed and may be useful in the control of certain virus diseases such as prophylaxis against influenza (type 2).

Human immunoglobulin

Normal human immunoglobulin (human gammaglobulin) has been used to produce passive immunisation against such infections as measles, rubella, infective hepatitis, paralytic poliomyelitis and other conditions. With the advances made in the active immunisation for some of these diseases the need for passive immunisation has become less. This substance is administered by intramuscular injection. The immunoglobulins have been assessed and identified and are made up mainly of IgG, IgA and IgM; very small amounts of IgD and IgE are also present. IgE levels are raised in allergic situations. In the newborn there is a high level of IgG transmitted from the mother which rapidly falls and then slowly increases; the other immunoglobulins are low in the newborn. The use of human immunoglobulin is valuable in the different syndromes of deficiencies of these globulins such as the rare condition of agammaglobulinaemia (Bruton's disease); this disease is transmitted as an X-linked condition.

Specific human immunoglobulin preparations prepared from the plasma of convalescent or recently immunised individuals are available against tetanus and vaccinia (useful in the treatment of smallpox vaccination complications). Another specific preparation is anti-D immunoglobulin (Rhesus factor) used in the prevention of haemolytic disease of the newborn due to Rhesus factor incompatibility; this is discussed in another section of this book.

Appendix I

Temperature equivalents

Centigrade degrees	Fahrenheit degrees
0	32
10	50
20	68
25	77
27	80·6
30	86
35	95
36	96·8
37	98·6
38	100·4
39	102·2
40	104
100	212

To convert Centigrade (Celsius) to Fahrenheit multiply by 9/5 and add 32.

To convert Fahrenheit to Centigrade (Celsius) subtract 32 and multiply by 5/9.

Weights and measures

Metric

1 gram (g)	= 1000 milligrams (mg)
1 kilogram (kg)	= 1000 grams
1 litre	= 1000 millilitres (ml)

Imperial

1 drachm	= 60 grains (gr) (Apothecary)
1 ounce	= 8 drachms = 480 grains (Apothecary)
1 fluid drachm	= 60 minims
1 fluid ounce	= 8 fluid drachms = 480 minims
1 pint	= 20 fluid ounces

Approximate dosage equivalents

Weights

1 kilogram (kg)	approximately = 2·2 pounds (lb)
1 gram (g)	approximately = 15 grains
1 grain (gr)	approximately = 64 milligrams (mg)
1 ounce (oz)	approximately = 30 grams

Fluid measures

1 millilitre (ml)	approximately = 16 minims
1 fluid ounce	approximately = 30 ml (28·4123 ml)
1 pint	approximately = 550 ml (568·2454 ml)
1 litre	approximately = 35 fl oz

The use of SI units in laboratories

Système International d'Unités (SI) is an international system based on the metre, kilogram, second and mole, and providing a system of units for different branches of science. It has led to the presentation of quantities and units in a uniform method. The amount of a substance is named on the SI system as mole with the symbol 'mol' being used; millimole is designated as mmol and micromole as μmol. In a similar way mass is designated as kilogram (kg), time as second (s), length as metre (m), electric current as ampere (A), and there are others of little interest in medicine. The unit of volume is the litre and the amount of a substance in concentration is designated as mole per litre (mol/l). The concentration of a mass is· designated as kilograms per litre (kg/l) and grams per litre (g/l). In practice the amount of a substance or its molar concentration is used for certain chemical substances and an example of a laboratory report for plasma urea as a normal range would be 2·5 to 6·5 mmol/l. The following are some important normal ranges in SI units in commonly used laboratory investigations:

Blood pH	7·35 to 7·45
Blood P_{CO_2}	4·5 to 6·1 kPa (kilopascal)
Standard bicarbonate	22 to 26 mmol/l
Base excess	± 2 mmol/l
Blood P_{O_2}	11·5 to 15·0 kPa
Alkaline phosphatase	150–470 i.u./l (children) (method according to T. U. Hausamen *et al.*)
Albumin	37 to 53 g/l
Amylase	70 to 300 i.u./l at 37°C (method of M. Ceska *et al.*)
Bilirubin (total)	2 to 15 μmol/l (300 μmol/l is approximately equivalent to 18 mg/100 ml)

Calcium	2·20 to 2·63 mmol/l
Chloride	95 to 105 mmol/l
Cholesterol (total)	4·0 to 5·2 mmol/l
Cortisol	100 to 600 mmol/l (peak value between 0800 to 1000 hours, lowest level around midnight)
Creatinephosphokinase (CPK)	up to 50 i.u./l at 25°C
Creatinine	60 to 120 μmol/l
Faecal fat	less than 4·5 g/day
Glucose (fasting) (blood)	3·5 to 5·5 mmol/l
Globulins	20 to 35 g/l
Lead (blood)	less than 1·7 μmol/l
Magnesium	0·78 to 1·03 mmol/l
Osmolality	270 to 285 mOsm/kg
Phosphate (inorganic)	Neonates 1·20 to 2·78 mmol/l
	Children 1·29 to 1·78 mmol/l
Proteins (total)	62 to 82 g/l
Salicylate	0 mmol/l (the therapeutic level is usually 1·5 to 2·2 mmol/l)
Sodium	136 to 148 mmol/l
Sweat sodium	less than 60 mmol/l
Transaminase, AST (SGOT)	5 to 17 i.u./l at 25°C
Urea	2·5 to 6·5 mmol/l
Uric acid	0·06 to 0·24 mmol/l (children)

Serum phenobarbitone—therapeutic level (old terminology) 10 to 20 μg/ml

Serum phenytoin (Epanutin)—therapeutic level (old terminology) 5 to 20 μg/ml

Appendix II

Composition of human milk (approximate)

Protein	1·25%
	(Lactalbumin 2 parts and casein 1 part)
Fat	3·5%
Carbohydrate (lactose)	7·25% plus water
Salts	0·2%
Calorific value	70 kilocalories per 100 ml

Composition of cow's milk (approximate)

Protein	3·5%
	(Lactalbumin 1 part and casein 5 parts)
Fat	3·5%
Carbohydrate	4·5% plus water
Salts	0·7%
Calorific value	70 kilocalories per 100 ml

4 g of sugar provides 15 calories.

Useful doses

Ampicillin (*Penbritin, Polycillin, Omnipen*). Under 40 kg 50 to 100 mg per kg bodyweight daily in four divided doses orally or by injection; over 40 kg and adults 1 to 2 g daily in divided doses.

Atropine (preoperative). Up to 1 year 0·1 to 0·2 mg, 1 to 5 years 0·2 to 0·3 mg, 6 to 12 years 0·3 to 0·5 mg, by subcutaneous injection.

Atropine methonitrate (*Eumydrin*). 0·6 per cent alcohol solution 1 minim 20 minutes before feeds orally; correspondingly larger doses for the *fresh* 1 in 1000 or 1 in 10,000 aqueous solutions (treatment for hypertrophic pyloric stenosis).

Cephaloridine (*Ceporin*). 30 to 50 mg per kg bodyweight daily in two or three divided doses by injection.

Chloramphenicol (*Chloromycetin*). Approximately 50 to 100 mg per kg bodyweight daily in divided doses, by mouth *but* much lower doses in premature and full-term newborn infants.

Chlorothiazide (Saluric). 20 mg per kg bodyweight daily in two oral doses.

Chlortetracycline (Aureomycin). 10 to 20 mg per kg bodyweight daily in divided doses, by mouth.

Demeclocycline (Ledermycin, Declomycin). 10 mg per kg bodyweight daily in divided doses, by mouth.

Deoxycycline (Vibramycin). Under 45 kg weight 4·4 mg per kg bodyweight daily in two doses with half the dose as maintenance; over 45 kg initial dose 200 mg in two doses then half the dose singly or in two doses daily orally.

Digitalis (digitalising dose). Digoxin (Lanoxin) 0·040 to 0·060 mg per kg bodyweight in divided doses by mouth. Digitoxin (Digitaline Nativelle) the same dosage for young children and 0·020 to 0·040 mg per kg bodyweight in divided doses by mouth for children over 2 years of age. Maintenance dose approximately one-quarter of the digitalising dose per day for digoxin and one-tenth for digitoxin. (Lower dosage in newborn and premature infants.)

Diphenhydramine (Benadryl). 4 mg per kg bodyweight daily in divided doses, by mouth.

Erythromycin (Ilotycin, Erythrocin). 20 to 40 mg per kg bodyweight daily in divided doses, by mouth.

Ethosuximide (Zarontin). Initially, under 6 years 0·25 g daily in divided doses orally and over 6 years 0·5 g orally in divided doses; the dosage may be increased if necessary by adding 0·25 g over four to seven days.

Glucagon. 0·025 mg per kg bodyweight as a single dose by injection.

Griseofulvin fine particle (Grisovin Fulcin). 10 mg per kg bodyweight daily in two to four doses orally.

Hydrochlorothiazide (HydroSaluric). One-tenth of the dose of chlorothiazide.

Isoniazid (INAH). 10 to 20 mg per kg bodyweight daily in divided doses, by mouth.

Kanamycin (Kantrex, Kannasyn). 15 mg per kg bodyweight daily in divided doses by intramuscular injection *but* lower doses in the newborn period.

Methicillin (Staphcillin, Celbenin, dimethoxyphenylpenicillin). 100 mg per kg bodyweight daily in divided doses by intramuscular injection.

Nalidixic acid (Negram). Over 1 month of age 50 mg per kg bodyweight daily orally in four divided doses.

Nitrofurantoin (Furadantin). 5 to 7 mg per kg bodyweight per day in divided doses, by mouth.

Nystatin (Nystan, Mycostatin). Newborn 400,000 units daily in four doses orally; older children 1 million units daily in four doses orally.

Oxytetracycline (Terramycin). 20 mg per kg bodyweight daily in divided doses, by mouth.

Paraldehyde. 0·15 ml per kg bodyweight per dose orally, rectally or by intramuscular injection. (If injected not to be used with a disposable syringe made of polystyrene, but may be given with a disposable syringe made of polypropylene or a glass syringe.)

Penicillin G. 25,000 to 50,000 units per kg bodyweight daily in four to six divided doses orally or by injection.

Phenobarbitone. For sedation 2 mg per kg bodyweight daily in three divided doses orally; as an anticonvulsant 3·5 mg per kg bodyweight for a single dose intramuscularly.

Phenoxymethylpenicillin (Penicillin V). 25,000 to 50,000 units per kg bodyweight daily in four divided doses orally.

Phenytoin (Epanutin, Dilantin). 3 to 8 mg per kg bodyweight daily orally in divided doses.

Sodium aminosalicylate (sodium PAS). 200 mg per kg bodyweight per day in divided doses, by mouth.

Streptomycin. 20 to 40 mg per kg bodyweight daily intramuscularly.

Tetracycline (Achromycin, Tetracyn, Polycycline, Tetrex). Approximately 20 mg per kg bodyweight daily in divided doses, by mouth.

Vincristine sulphate (Oncovin). 0·05 to 0·15 mg per kg bodyweight as a single weekly dose intravenously.

6-Mercaptopurine (Puri-nethol). 2·5 mg per kg bodyweight daily orally as a single dose.

For calculating drug dosage for children

In the past various formulae have been used for the calculation of the doses of drugs for infants and children and these included:

Young's formula:

$$\frac{\text{Age of the child (in years)}}{\text{Age of the child} + 12} \times \text{adult dose}$$

Clark's formula:

$$\frac{\text{Weight of the child (in pounds)}}{150} \times \text{adult dose}$$

(For children over 2 years of age)

Fried's formula:

$$\frac{\text{Age of the child (in months)}}{150} \times \text{adult dose}$$

(For infants under 2 years of age)

Dilling's formula:

$$\frac{\text{Age of the child}}{20} \times \text{adult dose}$$

Dosage scales for children are varied in relation to bodyweight and surface area. An appropriate method based more on surface area is the percentage method as outlined by Catzel. With this approach the concept of a basic adult dose is used. This is varied according to the age and weight and therefore the surface area of the child by calculating the percentage of the adult dose on the basis of the surface area of the child at the appropriate age.

Appendix III

Questions set at the Final State Examination for the Part of the Register for Sick Children's Nurses

(Reproduced by permission of the General Nursing Council for
England and Wales)

January 1972

(1964 Experimental Syllabus)

All Aspects of Nursing Care and Treatment of Sick Children

(Morning)

1. Give a detailed account of the nursing care and management of a 6-year-old child in status epilepticus.

2. Write short notes on four of the following: (a) care of the umbilicus in the newborn; (b) hazards of incubator nursing; (c) treatment of choanal atresia; (d) feeding of infants with micrognathia; (e) treatment of moniliasis (thrush).

3. (a) Describe the structure and function of lymph nodes. (b) List the causes of enlarged lymph nodes in the neck. (c) Describe the nursing care of a 5-year-old girl receiving radiotherapy for a cerebral tumour.

4. There has been an outbreak of gastroenteritis in the infants' ward of your hospital. (a) List the possible causative agents. (b) What steps would be taken to prevent the spread of infection? (c) Discuss the detailed nursing care and medical treatment of the affected infants.

5. (a) Give the age and range of the following milestones in childhood: (i) smiling; (ii) sitting up unsupported; (iii) saying single words meaningfully; (iv) dressing himself. (b) What factors may prevent a child reaching his milestones at the correct time?

6. What advice would you give to a mother whose child is being discharged with: (a) eczema; (b) a urinary diversion; (c) a ventriculo-atrial shunt (Holter valve)?

7. Write an essay on child abuse ('battered baby' syndrome).

(Afternoon)

1. (a) Describe the signs and symptoms of acute appendicitis in a 7-year-old child. (b) What are the complications of this condition? (c) Give a detailed account of the postoperative care of a child with generalised peritonitis.

2. What are the dangers of the following practical procedures and how may they be avoided: (a) a blood transfusion; (b) continuous urinary drainage with a self-retaining catheter; (c) a rectal washout; (d) an underwater drain from the pleural cavity?

3. (a) Describe the heart with the aid of a labelled diagram. (b) List some of the commoner congenital heart defects. (c) Describe the nursing and medical care of an infant in congestive heart failure.

4. Discuss the hazards of nursing sick children in adult wards.

5. (a) Describe in detail the effects of prolonged vomiting due to pyloric stenosis. (b) Give an account of the pre- and postoperative care of an infant having a pyloromyotomy (Ramstedt's operation).

6. Write short notes on four of the following: (a) torticollis; (b) strawberry naevus (cavernous haemangioma); (c) talipes equino-varus; (d) umbilical hernia; (e) a convergent squint.

7. A newborn baby is admitted with an oesophageal atresia and tracheo-oesophageal fistula. Discuss the following: (a) the early recognition and diagnosis of this condition; (b) the preoperative nursing care; (c) how the baby may be fed in the first week following operation; (d) the help and advice given to the parents.

June 1972

(1964 Experimental Syllabus)

All Aspects of Nursing Care and Treatment of Sick Children

(Morning)

1. (a) What are the signs and symptoms of meningococcal meningitis in a 6-year-old girl? (b) Give a detailed account of the nursing care and medical treatment of such a child.

2. Describe how you would assist the doctor in the following procedures: (a) jugular venepuncture for collection of a specimen of blood; (b) lumbar puncture for the collection of a specimen of cerebrospinal fluid from a 4-year-old child; (c) examination of the ears of a 2-year-old child; (d) examination of the fundi for the presence of papilloedema in a 10-year-old boy.

3. A 3-month-old infant requires an intramuscular injection of 0·15 mg (150 micrograms) of digoxin. (a) Describe how you would administer this dose from a vial containing 0·5 mg (500 micrograms) in 2 ml. (b) What are the indications for use of digoxin? By what other routes may it be administered and what are the side-effects of digoxin?

4. (a) Briefly describe how proteins are digested, absorbed and utilised in the body. (b) How would you calculate the 24-hour feed requirements of an 8-week-old infant who weighed 5½ lb (2·5 kg) at birth and is being artificially fed? (c) What added supplements should be given?

5. (a) Enumerate the signs and symptoms of severe bronchiolitis in a young infant. (b) Give a detailed account of the nursing care and medical treatment of such an infant.

6. (a) Give an account of the cycle of events taking place in the heart during a normal beat (cardiac cycle). (b) What would lead you to suspect that a child has suffered circulatory and respiratory arrest? (c) Describe your activities prior to arrival of the medical staff.

7. Write short notes on three of the following: (a) pseudo hypertrophic muscular dystrophy; (b) haemophilia; (c) mucoviscidosis (cystic fibrosis); (d) phenylketonuria. What have these diseases in common? What general advice may be given to the parents of these children?

(Afternoon)

1. (a) Describe, with the aid of a diagram, the gross structure of the kidney. A child aged 6 years has suspected right hydronephrosis. (b) List the investigations that will be carried out to confirm this diagnosis. (c) Describe in detail the postoperative nursing care for this patient following a right pyeloplasty.

2. A 10-year-old boy has sustained a severe head injury resulting in left hemiplegia. Discuss: (a) the rehabilitation in the ward; and (b) the long-term management of this patient on his return home.

3. A junior nurse is to remove sutures for the first time. What are your responsibilities as a senior nurse in this situation?

4. Write a short account of four of the following: (a) Perthes' disease (osteochondritis); (b) congenital cataract; (c) nocturnal enuresis; (d) acute maxillary sinusitis; (e) impetigo.

5. Discuss the importance of play in child development. What special provisions for play can be made for the sick child?

6. (a) Describe the clotting process of blood.

A boy of 18 months is to be admitted for the repair of a complete cleft palate. (b) What advice will be given to the parents prior to admission? (c) Describe the special nursing care required to avoid postoperative complications.

7. A newborn baby weighing 2 kg (4·4 lb) has a diaphragmatic hernia. Write an account of: (a) the preoperative care; (b) the postoperative nursing care.

October 1972

All Aspects of Nursing Care and Treatment of Sick Children

(Morning)

1. Four days following admission, a 3-year-old child in a children's ward develops measles. (a) List the signs, symptoms and complications of measles. (b) Explain why some of his contacts may not develop the infection. (c) What nursing and medical measures should be taken to prevent the spread of infection?

2. You are in charge of the ward during the absence of Sister. What would your action be in the following situations: (a) an 8-year-old girl being admitted to the ward has pediculi capitis (head lice); (b) a mother wishes to take home her very ill child against medical advice; (3) a 2-year-old boy falls out of his cot?

3. (a) What are the symptoms and signs of diabetes mellitus in childhood? Explain why these occur. (b) Discuss the management of a 7-year-old girl in a diabetic coma (hyperglycaemic coma) during the first 48 hours following admission.

4. List the actions, indications for use and side-effects of four of the following: (a) phenytoin; (b) cortisone; (c) sulphadimidine; (d) sodium salicylate; (e) methotrexate.

5. Give a detailed account of the nursing care and observation of a newborn infant weighing 1·25 kg (2 lb 12 oz).

6. Write notes on three of the following: (a) primary complex (tuberculosis); (b) thrombocytopenia; (c) disaccharide intolerance; (d) rheumatoid arthritis (Still's disease).

7. (a) Describe how atmospheric oxygen reaches the tissues. (b) For what reasons may a tracheostomy be performed? (c) Describe the local care of a tracheostomy during the first 48 hours following operation.

(Afternoon)

1. (a) With the aid of a diagram, describe the structure of the small intestine. (b) What are the clinical features that would lead you to suspect that George, aged 1 year, is suffering from acute intussusception? (c) Discuss the possible methods of treatment. (d) Describe the preoperative management of this patient.

2. Discuss the statement 'the patient and his relatives are reassured'.

3. A 1-month-old baby in cardiac failure is admitted to the ward. (a) 0·125 mg of digoxin is ordered to be given. Describe how you would calculate this dose from a vial containing 0·5 mg (500 micrograms) in 2 ml. (b) Discuss the feeding of this baby.

4. A 10-year-old boy has sustained severe burns of his right thigh and groin. Describe (a) the first-aid treatment; and (b) the subsequent treatment and nursing care of this patient.

5. (a) Write an account of the functions of the lymphatic system. (b) List the

complications that may occur after a tonsillectomy and adenoidectomy. (c) Describe how these complications may be avoided, recognised and treated if necessary.

6. Write a short account of four of the following: (a) meconium ileus; (b) torticollis; (c) phimosis; (d) convergent squint; (e) psoriasis.

7. A 4-year-old girl with a repaired meningomyelocele has had a urinary diversion and is to be discharged. (a) What arrangements should be made prior to her discharge? (b) What facilities are available in the community for her care at home?

January 1973

All Aspects of Nursing Care and Treatment of Sick Children

(Morning)

1. (a) Describe the appearance of a 9-month-old obese infant with severe bronchiolitis. (b) Give a detailed account of his nursing care and medical treatment.

2. A 2-year-old child is admitted having swallowed a large quantity of iron tablets. (a) What immediate care would this child require in the accident and emergency department? (b) Describe his subsequent care and treatment following admission to the ward.

3. In three of the following—(a) a 1-year-old for jejunal biopsy, (b) a 7-year-old for cardiac catheterisation, (c) a 10-year-old girl for micturating cystogram, (d) a 5-year-old for barium enema—describe: (i) your preparation of the child; (ii) the procedure (brief outline only); (iii) the significance of the observations made following the child's return to the ward.

4. Two days following appendicectomy with drainage, a 7-year-old boy in a surgical ward is found to have Sonne dysentery. (a) What immediate precautions should be taken to prevent the spread of infection? (b) Give a detailed account of his subsequent nursing care and treatment.

5. The alternative to home care is to admit the sick child to hospital. What facilities should be provided to help alleviate the adverse effects of such an admission?

6. (a) What are the functions of the liver? (b) List the common causes of pathological jaundice in infancy. (c) A newborn infant weighing 2 kg (4·4 lb) develops physiological jaundice. What nursing care and treatment may this infant require?

7. 'The wealth of a nation is invested in the health of its children.' Discuss this statement under the following headings: (a) breast feeding; (b) immunisation; (c) the school health service.

(Afternoon)

1. (a) Describe the preparation of an infant for a scalp vein infusion. (b) What are the dangers of such an infusion? (c) What measures are taken to avoid these complications?

2. A 3-year-old child is admitted for adenoidectomy. (a) Describe the management of this patient during his stay in hospital. (b) List the constituents of blood. (c) Describe the clotting process.

3. Write a short account of four of the following: (a) the use of glasses in the treatment of convergent squint; (b) the reasons for bone marrow puncture; (c) the care of the ear following myringotomy; (d) the care of a pedicle graft; (e) the treatment of phenylketonuria.

4. Discuss how the needs of the mentally handicapped child are met in hospital and in the community.

5. A very ill 7-year-old child is admitted to the ward with suspected osteomyelitis of his right femur. (a) Describe, with the aid of a labelled diagram, a long bone. Indicate the possible site of infection. (b) Discuss the possible treatment. (c) Describe the nursing care during the acute stage of his illness.

6. (a) Why is premedication given before an anaesthetic? (b) Give examples of

four drugs used for this purpose and state their route of administration. (c) What information should the ward nurse have available for the anaesthetist when accompanying patients to the operating theatre?

7. (a) Compare and contrast the signs and symptoms of raised intracranial pressure in: (i) a 6-week-old infant; (ii) a 6-year-old child. (b) Describe the nursing care of an infant following a ventriculo-atrial shunt.

June 1973

All Aspects of Nursing Care and Treatment of Sick Children

(Morning)

1. A 6-year-old boy is admitted in status asthmaticus. (a) What would you observe about this child's appearance and behaviour? (b) What drugs may be prescribed? (c) Detail his nursing care during the acute stage of illness.

2. (a) Describe the structure and functions of the small intestine. (b) With these functions in mind describe: (i) coeliac disease; (ii) cystic fibrosis (mucoviscidosis); (iii) disaccharide intolerance.

3. A 10-year-old girl is admitted to the ward with suspected acute leukaemia. (a) What investigations may be made to confirm the diagnosis? (b) What medical treatment may be prescribed? (c) Describe the nursing care of this child in the terminal stage of illness.

4. Write notes on two of the following: (a) Rhesus incompatibility; (b) intravenous alimentation (feeding); (c) neonatal hypoglycaemia.

5. A 3-year-old boy is admitted for the day for circumcision. (a) For what reasons may this operation be performed? (b) What instructions would be given to the mother prior to his admission to the ward? (c) Discuss the role of the mother during his stay in hospital. (d) What advice would be given prior to his discharge home?

6. (a) Describe the local features of inflammation. (b) What effect may an area of localised inflammation have on the body as a whole? (c) Discuss the nursing care and medical treatment of a toddler with a large submandibular abscess.

7. Discuss the factors which have led to a decline in the incidence of infectious diseases in this country during the last thirty years.

(Afternoon)

1. A 4-year-old boy is admitted with intestinal obstruction thought to be due to adhesions. Describe in detail: (a) the preoperative care; (b) the postoperative nursing care.

2. (a) Draw a labelled diagram showing the structure of the skin. (b) List the functions of the skin. (c) Describe the management, in hospital and at home, of a girl aged 15 months with infantile eczema.

3. How would you explain three of the following medical terms to parents: (a) cerebral palsy; (b) hydrocephalus; (c) ileal conduit; (d) imperforate anus?

4. A newborn baby is admitted with an oesophageal atresia and tracheo-oesophageal fistula. Describe: (a) the clinical manifestations; (b) the preoperative care; (c) the nursing care following primary anastomosis of the oesophagus and closure of the fistula.

5. (a) Describe the formation of urine. (b) State how you will collect a clean specimen of urine from: (i) a girl aged 3 months; (ii) a boy aged 7 years. (c) List the renal function tests.

6. Give a detailed account of the care of a 12-year-old child undergoing long-term treatment in hospital for an orthopaedic condition of your choice.

7. (a) What factors influence child development? (b) When would you expect the following milestones to be reached: (i) sitting unaided; (ii) saying single words meaningfully; (iii) drinking from a cup; (iv) being dry at night?

October 1973
All Aspects of Nursing Care and Treatment of Sick Children

(Morning)

1. An infant in a children's ward develops diarrhoea. Discuss the management of this situation.

2. (a) Explain why ketosis develops in untreated diabetes mellitus. (b) Describe the nursing care and medical treatment of an 8-year-old girl admitted to the ward in a diabetic (hyperglycaemic) coma.

3. Choose any one child you have nursed who has ingested a toxic substance and describe: (a) his immediate care in the accident and emergency department; (b) his subsequent care and treatment following admission to the ward; (c) the advice given to the parents prior to his discharge home.

4. (a) List the complications to which an infant of low birth weight is prone. (b) Discuss the role of the nurse in the early recognition or prevention of five of the complications you have listed.

5. Answer either A or B. A. (a) With the aid of a diagram, describe the structure and function of the ear. (b) What are the causes of deafness in childhood? (c) Discuss the education and care required by deaf children. B. (a) With the aid of a diagram, describe the structure and function of the eye. (b) What are the causes of blindness in childhood? (c) Discuss the education and care required by blind children.

6. 'Job or patient assignment.' Discuss the advantages and disadvantages of each to: (a) the child; (b) his parents; (c) the nurse.

7. Write short notes on four of the following: (a) torticollis; (b) hypospadias; (c) undescended testes; (d) nocturnal enuresis; (e) Perthes' disease.

(Afternoon)

1. A 3-year-old girl has a right nephroblastoma (Wilms' tumour). Describe: (a) the preoperative care; (b) the postoperative care following right nephrectomy.

2. (a) With the aid of a labelled diagram, describe the flow of blood through the heart. (b) What are the causes of heart failure in the first year of life? (c) Give a detailed account of the nursing care and medical treatment of a 5-month-old infant in heart failure.

3. Describe the immediate and long-term management of the relatives in the following situations: (a) a 10-month-old baby admitted with 40 per cent scalds sustained in the home; (b) a 2-year-old boy admitted with pneumonia as a complication of cystic fibrosis (mucoviscidosis).

4. (a) With the aid of a diagram, describe the structure and functions of the small intestine. (b) List the causes of dysfunction of this part of the gut that may arise in the first year of life. (c) Describe the investigations that may be carried out in such cases.

5. Describe how you would prepare the patient and assist the doctor in the following situations: (a) an infant who is having a venepuncture; (b) a 3-year-old child who is having a lumbar puncture; (c) a 10-year-old girl who is having a rectal examination.

6. Choose one infant you have nursed who has undergone surgery during the first week of life. Describe: (a) the condition you have chosen; (b) the specific postoperative care; (c) the education of the parents prior to the baby's discharge home.

7. A 10-year-old boy has been admitted with head and spinal injuries following a road traffic accident. (a) List the observations that should be made. (b) Discuss the significance of these observations and any action that might have to be taken.

January 1974

All Aspects of Nursing Care and Treatment of Sick Children

(Morning)

1. Give a detailed account of the pre- and postoperative nursing care of a 15-month-old boy admitted to the ward for the repair of his complete cleft-palate.

2. In three of the following—(a) circumcision, (b) adenoidectomy, (c) lengthening of Achilles tendon, (d) myringotomy—describe: (i) the reasons for which each operation is performed; (ii) the specific postoperative management; (iii) the advice given to the mother prior to her child's discharge from hospital.

3. A girl aged 6 years is suspected to be suffering from primary tuberculous lung infection. Discuss the total management of this situation.

4. Discuss the role of the paediatric nurse in two of the following: (a) the storage and administration of drugs; (b) ensuring the safety of her patients; (c) providing opportunities for play.

5. (a) Describe the formation of urine. (b) Discuss the nursing care and medical treatment of an 8-year-old boy who is admitted to hospital with marked signs of nephrotic syndrome.

6. Describe a suitable feeding regime for the following infants giving reasons for your choice of food, times of feeding, and methods of administration. (a) a 1-month-old infant who weighed 1 kg (2·2 lb) at birth; (b) a 4-month-old boy who weighed 3·4 kg (7·5 lb) at birth; (c) a 9-month-old girl who now weighs 10 kg (22 lb).

7. (a) Describe the formation, functions and destruction of erythrocytes (red blood corpuscles). (b) Discuss the causes, clinical manifestations and treatment of two of the following: (i) sickle-cell anaemia; (ii) aplastic anaemia; (iii) thalassaemia; (iv) spherocytosis (familial acholuric jaundice).

(Afternoon)

1. (a) List the possible causes of convulsions during the first two years of life. (b) Describe, in detail, the total care of a patient with one condition that you have mentioned.

2. A 7-year-old boy is admitted to the ward following the explosion of fireworks in his trouser pocket. (a) Describe, with the aid of a labelled diagram, the structure of the skin. (b) List the functions of the skin. (c) Describe the nursing care and management during his first 48 hours in hospital.

3. Discuss the role of the mother in a children's ward.

4. Choose one infant you have nursed who has undergone surgery during the first week of life. Describe: (a) the condition you have chosen; (b) the specific post-operative care; (c) the education of the parents prior to the baby's discharge home.

5. An 11-year-old boy is admitted to the ward with a fractured shaft of femur following a fall whilst playing football. (a) Describe, with the aid of a labelled diagram, a long bone. (b) Discuss the total care of this boy during his stay in hospital.

6. A 9-year-old girl is admitted to the ward for terminal care. (a) What measures may be taken to relieve the child's pain and anxiety? (b) How may the family be helped and supported during this time?

7. What would lead you to suspect the following and what action would you take in each instance: (a) a child is bleeding 6 hours following tonsillectomy; (b) a child is developing measles; (c) a child has infested hair?

June 1974

All Aspects of Nursing Care and Treatment of Sick Children

(Morning)

1. (a) What are the signs and symptoms of meningococcal meningitis in an

18-month-old boy? (b) Give a detailed account of the nursing care and medical treatment of this child.

2. (a) List five causes of dyspnoea in the first seven days of life. (b) What may lead you to suspect that an infant of low birth weight is developing respiratory distress syndrome? (c) Give a detailed account of the nursing care and medical treatment of such an infant.

3. (a) With the aid of a labelled diagram describe the hip joint. (b) How is congenital dislocation of the hip diagnosed in infancy? (c) How may this condition be treated? (d) Describe the special care required by an infant in an abduction splint.

4. Discuss the role of (a) the nurse in hospital, (b) the health visitor, in the early detection and management of child abuse ('battered baby' syndrome).

5. (a) Describe the clotting process of blood. (b) Give a detailed account of the total care and treatment of a 6-year-old girl with either (i) idiopathic thrombocytopenic purpura, or (ii) Henoch-Schönlein purpura.

6. How would you explain the necessity for a special diet and gain the co-operation of a child in this respect in three of the following: (a) a 6-year-old boy with acute glomerular nephritis; (b) an 11-year-old girl weighing 70 kg (11 stones); (c) a 5-year-old boy with 35 per cent burns; (d) a 7-year-old girl with diabetes mellitus?

7. Write notes on the causes and treatment of three of the following: (a) moniliasis (thrush); (b) anorexia nervosa; (c) stridor; (d) napkin rash; (e) hypoglycaemia.

(Afternoon)

1. A 6-year-old girl has a persistent (patent) ductus arteriosus. (a) Draw a labelled diagram of the heart and great vessels illustrating this defect. (b) Describe the postoperative care of this child following ligation of the ductus.

2. How would you explain four of the following conditions to a junior nurse: (a) strabismus; (b) syndactyly; (c) otorrhoea; (d) encopresis; (e) paronychia.

3. A 4-year-old boy with hypospadias is seen in the outpatient department. (a) How can the nurse help the parents to prepare the child for admission to hospital? (b) Describe his care from arrival at hospital until he is taken to the operating theatre.

4. (a) What are the functions of the hormones produced by the adrenal cortex? (b) Enumerate five conditions in childhood for which steroid therapy may be of value. (c) Describe the side-effects of prolonged steroid therapy.

5. Write an essay on the significance of observations relating to the physical, emotional and social wellbeing of a toddler.

6. A 10-year-old girl is admitted to the ward with a suspected cerebral tumour. (a) List the investigations which may be required to confirm the diagnosis. (b) Describe either (i) the specific nursing care of this child following craniotomy, or (ii) the specific nursing care of this child receiving radiotherapy. (c) How may the parents be helped in this situation?

7. A 2-month-old baby boy has a right inguinal hernia. He is admitted as a day case for surgery. (a) What is an inguinal hernia? (b) Describe the management of this patient. (c) List the other sites of herniae.

September 1974

All Aspects of Nursing Care and Treatment of Sick Children

(Morning)

1. Choose one infant you have nursed who has undergone major surgery during the first week of life. Describe: (a) the condition you have chosen; (b) the specific postoperative care; (c) the education of the parents prior to the infant's discharge home.

2. A child aged 10 years suffering from leukaemia is readmitted to the ward at

the end of a period of remission. (a) How would you describe the nature of this illness to a junior colleague? (b) Discuss the nursing care in the terminal stage of illness. (c) How may the family be helped and supported during this time?

3. (a) Show how you would work out the feed requirements of a normal healthy infant aged 6 weeks, whose birth weight was 3 kg (approximately 7 lb) who is to be bottle-fed. (b) Describe in detail how you would make up one feed for this infant. (c) What advice would you give to a mother regarding the introduction of mixed feeding?

4. A girl aged 4 years with spina bifida is admitted to the ward for either (i) the construction of an ileal conduit, or (ii) a psoas muscle transplant. (a) Describe the pre- and postoperative nursing care of this child. (b) What advice would be given to the parents prior to her discharge home?

5. What precautions are taken to ensure that small children receive the appropriate drug dosage? Illustrate your answer by describing how you would administer an oral dose of 0·125 mg (125 micrograms) of elixir of digoxin from a stock bottle containing 0·05 mg (50 micrograms) in 1 ml.

6. (a) Draw a labelled diagram to show the structure of the skin and list its functions. (b) Give a detailed account of the nursing care and treatment of a 3-year-old boy admitted with either (i) severe eczema, or (ii) syndactyly (webbed fingers).

7. Discuss the provisions made for mentally handicapped children and the relative advantages and disadvantages of such children being cared for in institutions or in their own homes.

(Afternoon)

1. A 6-week-old infant is admitted to the ward with gastroenteritis. (a) What are the aims of treatment? (b) Describe in detail the total care of this infant. (c) What help and advice should be given to the parents?

2. A 7-year-old boy is admitted to the ward with newly diagnosed diabetes mellitus. (a) List the possible symptoms and signs. (b) Explain why these symptoms and signs occur. (c) Outline his treatment in hospital and describe how you would prepare the child and his parents to cope successfully with this condition in the future.

3. Write notes on three of the following: (a) choanal atresia; (b) meconium ileus; (c) coarctation of the aorta; (d) galactosaemia.

4. A happy ward atmosphere is conducive to good standards of nursing care and the wellbeing of the patients. Discuss this statement.

5. (a) Why is the efficient functioning of the kidneys essential for health? (b) Describe in detail either (i) the total care of an 18-month-old girl undergoing peritoneal dialysis, or (ii) the total care of an 18-month-old girl with acute pyelonephritis.

6. A 10-year-old boy has been admitted with a fractured base of skull following a road traffic accident. (a) List the observations that should be made. (b) Discuss the significance of these observations and any action that might have to be taken.

7. (a) For what reasons may a tracheostomy be performed? (b) Describe in detail the treatment and care required by a patient who has had a tracheostomy performed for any one cause you have mentioned. State the age of the patient and relate your answer to this.

February 1975

All Aspects of Nursing Care and Treatment of Sick Children

(Morning)

1. Describe the total care and management of a 3-year-old boy admitted to hospital for treatment of a perforated appendix.

2. (a) What is immunity and how may it be acquired? (b) List the diseases against which children are commonly immunised. (c) Give an account of the total care

required by a 14-month-old boy admitted to hospital with a severe attack of either whooping cough or measles.

3. Describe a suitable feeding regime for the following infants giving reasons for your choice of food, times of feeding and methods of administration. (a) a 1-week-old infant who weighed 1 kg (2·2 lb) at birth; (b) a 3-month-old boy who weighed 3·4 kg (7·5 lb) at birth; (c) a 9-month-old girl who now weighs 10 kg (22 lb).

4. (a) Give an account of the cycle of events taking place in the heart during one beat. (b) What would lead you to suspect that a child had suffered a cardiac and respiratory arrest? What would you do until the arrival of the resuscitation team?

5. An 8-year-old girl has been in hospital for six months with a residual paraplegia following spinal injury. She is to be discharged home. Discuss: (a) the problems which may arise within the family (parents, older brother and new baby); (b) the hospital and community services available to help in this situation.

6. (a) Describe the absorption of foodstuffs in the small intestine. (b) What is coeliac disease, how is it recognised and how is the diagnosis confirmed? (c) Outline the dietary management of this condition.

7. What would you teach a junior nurse about the importance of ensuring that children in hospital receive adequate: (a) sleep and rest; (b) play and education; (c) contact with home?

(Afternoon)

1. A boy aged 5 years is admitted to the ward for removal of tonsils and adenoids. (a) Describe the total preoperative care of this child including the part played by the parents. (b) List the postoperative observations that should be made until the child is discharged home. (c) Discuss the significance of these observations and any action that might have to be taken.

2. (a) What may prevent a child reaching his milestones at the correct age? (b) Discuss the function of child assessment units in determining the future care of handicapped children.

3. (a) Describe a typical synovial joint. (b) Give an account of the nursing care and management of either (i) a 7-year-old girl admitted to hospital with rheumatoid arthritis (Still's disease) or (ii) a 7-year-old sufferer of haemophilia admitted to hospital with haemarthrosis of his left knee.

4. In three of the following—(a) pediculosis, (b) moniliasis (thrush), (c) scabies, (d) threadworms—describe: (i) how you would recognise the condition; (ii) the specific treatment; (iii) the measures taken to prevent the spread of the infestation or infection.

5. (a) How is the body temperature maintained at a fairly constant level? (b) Describe the nursing care and treatment of a 2-week-old infant admitted to hospital with a temperature of 30°C (86°F).

6. (a) What is hydronephrosis and how may the condition arise? (b) What investigations may be carried out to confirm this diagnosis? (c) Describe the pre- and postoperative care of a 10-year-old girl admitted to hospital for an operation for unilateral hydronephrosis.

7. A 10-month-old infant with head injuries is admitted to the ward for observation. (a) Describe the total care of this infant for the 24 hours after admission. (b) What might lead you to suspect that the injuries are non-accidental?

June 1975

All Aspects of Nursing Care and Treatment of Sick Children

(Morning)

1. (a) List the micro-organisms which may cause meningitis in infancy and childhood. (b) Give a detailed account of the nursing care and medical treatment of

an 18-month-old child suffering from a meningeal infection caused by one of the micro-organisms you have listed.

2. There has been an outbreak of gastroenteritis in the infants' ward of your hospital. (a) What steps should be taken to prevent the spread of this infection? (b) Discuss the detailed nursing care and medical treatment of the affected infants.

3. Choose any one child you have nursed who has ingested a toxic substance and describe: (a) his immediate care in the accident and emergency department; (b) his subsequent care and treatment following admission to the ward; (c) the advice given to the parents prior to his discharge home.

4. What precautions should be taken to ensure that small children receive the appropriate drug dosage? Illustrate your answer by describing how you would help to prepare your junior colleagues to accept this responsibility.

5. (a) Describe the mechanics of normal respiration. (b) Give a detailed account of either (i) the total care of an 8-year-old boy in status asthmaticus or (ii) the total care of an 8-year-old boy requiring intermittent positive pressure ventilation.

6. Obesity is a problem in our affluent society. (a) Discuss the ways in which infants and small children can be protected from becoming overweight. (b) Give a detailed account of the total management of a 14-year-old girl admitted to hospital weighing 90 kg (approximately 14 stones).

7. (a) Describe the circulation of blood through the heart. (b) List some of the more common congenital heart defects. (c) Describe the nursing care and medical treatment of an infant in congestive heart failure.

(Afternoon)

1. A girl aged 10 years sustained burns of the legs and lower trunk when her long party dress caught fire. (a) Describe, in detail, the management of this girl for the first 48 hours following admission to hospital. (b) How may the nurse: (i) help and support the distressed parents at this time; (ii) advise them on the part they can play in their daughter's recovery?

2. What nursing measures may be taken in three of the following situations: (a) when a 5-year-old boy with diabetes mellitus who has had insulin refuses breakfast; (b) when a 3-year-old girl, newly admitted to hospital, wakes crying in the night; (c) when a 6-year-old boy soils due to chronic constipation; (d) when a 4-year-old mentally handicapped child persistently bangs his head?

3. A 15-month-old boy is admitted to the ward for repair of cleft palate. (a) What specific preoperative preparation should this child and his mother receive? (b) Describe his nursing care from the time of operation until his discharge home.

4. What services are available to help parents to keep a child, who is both mentally and physically handicapped due to cerebral palsy, at home for as long as possible?

5. (a) Make a list of headings under which total nursing care may be described. (b) Using these headings, give an account of the total care of either (i) a premature infant who weighs 1·5 kg (3·3 lb) or (ii) a 2-day-old infant who has undergone repair of diaphragmatic hernia.

6. An 8-month-old infant is admitted with intussusception. (a) With reference to anatomy and physiology, describe how intussusception occurs. (b) Give an account of the preoperative management and postoperative care following reduction of the intussusception.

7. In three of the following—(a) circumcision, (b) adenoidectomy, (c) lengthening of Achilles tendon, (d) myringotomy—describe (i) the reasons for which each operation is performed; (ii) the specific postoperative management; (iii) the advice given to the mother prior to her child's discharge from hospital.

October 1975

All Aspects of Nursing Care and Treatment of Sick Children

(Morning)

1. (a) Describe the composition and functions of the blood. (b) Give an account of the total nursing care required by a 20-month-old girl receiving a blood transfusion for severe anaemia.

2. (a) List the common causes of convulsions in infancy and childhood. (b) State the detailed observations which you should make during a convulsion. (c) Name three drugs used to control convulsions. (d) What first-aid measures should you take when a 3-year-old child has a convulsion in a busy supermarket?

3. (a) With reference to anatomy and physiology, state the ways in which cystic fibrosis may present. (b) Describe the total nursing care and treatment of a 7-year-old boy with cystic fibrosis admitted with an acute chest infection.

4. A 12-year-old girl is admitted to hospital, newly diagnosed as having diabetes mellitus. (a) List the possible signs and symptoms. (b) Outline her medical and nursing treatment. (c) How would you prepare this adolescent girl and her parents to understand and manage her condition successfully?

5. (a) Describe the circulation and function of cerebrospinal fluid. (b) Give a detailed account of the postoperative nursing care of a 2-week-old infant following insertion of a ventriculo-atrial shunt. (c) What specific observations should the mother be taught to make to detect early complications?

6. How would you explain three of the following conditions and briefly outline the treatment to a junior nurse: (a) talipes equino-varus; (b) hypospadias; (c) phenyl-ketonuria; (d) persistent ductus arteriosus?

7. If you select this question answer either A or B. A (a) With the aid of a diagram describe the structure and function of the ear. (b) What are the causes of deafness in childhood? (c) Discuss the education and care required by deaf children.

B. (a) With the aid of a diagram describe the structure and function of the eye. (b) What are the causes of blindness in childhood? (c) Discuss the education and care required by blind children.

(Afternoon)

1. A 6-week-old boy baby is admitted to the ward with pyloric stenosis for Ramstedt's operation (pyloromyotomy). (a) List the signs of pyloric stenosis. (b) Explain, with reference to anatomy and physiology, why these signs occur. (c) Describe the preparation of this baby for surgery. (d) Discuss the postoperative feeding régime until his discharge home.

2. (a) List the reasons why tracheostomy may be performed. (b) Describe, in detail, the total care of any one patient you have nursed for the first 48 hours following tracheostomy. State the age and condition of the patient and relate your answer to this.

3. You are in charge of the ward. (a) What would lead you to suspect that a patient's wound is infected? (b) What action would you take in this situation? (c) What measures should be taken in a surgical ward to prevent cross-infection?

4. A 3-year-old girl has a right nephroblastoma (Wilms' tumour). She is admitted to the ward for nephrectomy and radiotherapy. (a) Describe either: (i) the nursing care of this child for the first 48 hours following surgery; or (ii) the nursing care of this child whilst receiving radiotherapy. (b) How may the parents be helped?

5. A 6-year-old child, severely physically handicapped by cerebral palsy, is admitted to the ward while his parents go on holiday. (a) What information do you need from the parents before they leave? (b) How would you minimise regression and help

the child to progress during his stay in hospital? (c) List the facilities and agencies available to help parents to continue to care for handicapped children at home.

6. A 10-year-old girl has been admitted to the ward with a fractured left femur which has been satisfactorily immobilised by skin traction. (a) With the aid of a labelled diagram, describe a long bone. (b) Describe, in detail, the total care of this girl whilst in hospital.

7. A 2-year-old boy has a right inguinal hernia. He is admitted as a day patient for surgery. (a) Describe the total preoperative care of this child including the part played by the parents. (b) Discuss the advantages and disadvantages of day surgery for this child and his family.

Questions set at the Final State Examination for the Parts of the Register for Sick Children's and General Nurses

October 1975

All Aspects of Nursing Care and Treatment of Patients

(Morning)

Section A

1. A girl aged 6 years is to be admitted to a ward with a provisional diagnosis of acute meningitis. (a) State briefly the special preparations you would make for the reception of this child in the ward and for the diagnostic investigations. (b) Give an account of the nursing care which the child may be given after diagnosis of acute meningitis has been confirmed. (c) What could the nursing staff do to help the parents while this child is in hospital?

2. How would you explain to an inexperienced nurse the possible reasons for three of the following and what would you advise her to do in each situation you have chosen: (a) a child aged 2 years has a temper tantrum when taken from the play group for essential treatment; (b) a toddler screams and struggles when the nurse tries to put him into the bath for the first time after his admission to the ward; (c) a convalescent girl aged 5 years persistently wets her bed at night; (d) a boy aged 10 years is found to have in his locker a number of articles taken from other children in the ward?

3. (a) What are the typical symptoms and signs of acute idiopathic intussusception in infancy? (b) Describe the nursing care of a child aged 10 months during the first 48 hours following laparotomy and reduction of an intussusception, mentioning the part played by the parents. (c) State briefly the dangers of delay in recognition and treatment of intussusception.

4. (a) Describe the normal action of the heart during one cardiac cycle. (b) List six possible clinical features of congenital heart disease in early infancy. (c) Give an account of the medical treatment and special nursing care which may be given to a baby aged 6 weeks admitted to hospital with signs of heart failure.

Section B

5. (a) Describe the structure of the bronchial tree, including the alveoli. (b) Give an account of the total care of a patient admitted to hospital in an acute attack of bronchial asthma. State the age of the patient you have chosen.

6. (a) List the possible complications of an open fracture. (b) What preoperative treatment and care would be given to a patient admitted to hospital with open fracture of tibia and fibula? (c) State the special observations the nurse should make on a patient who has had a plaster of Paris applied after reduction of such a fracture.

7. If you select this question, answer either A or B.

A. (a) Draw and label a diagram to show the structure of the eye-ball. (b) Give an account of the help available in the community for: (i) a blind child and his family; (ii) and a blind adult.

B. (a) Describe the physiology of hearing. (b) Discuss what can be done to help children and adults with hearing disability.

8. (a) Why may it be necessary for a tracheostomy to be performed? (b) Describe in detail the treatment and care required by a patient who has had a tracheostomy performed for any one cause you have mentioned. State the age of the patient and relate your answer to this.

(Afternoon)

Section A

1. (a) Describe the rectum and give an account of defaecation. (b) How would a patient be prepared for, and cared for, following the operation of haemorrhoidectomy?

2. If you select this question, answer either A or B.

A. (a) Write an account of the three stages of labour. (b) Describe the observations you would make and the care you would give to a mother during the first stage of labour.

B. A 70-year-old man, who lives alone, is admitted to the ward for operation for an enlarged prostate gland. (a) List the clinical features of an enlarged prostate gland. (b) Give an account of the postoperative care the patient may require. (c) What services are available to enable this patient to return home as soon as possible?

3. A middle-aged man, admitted to hospital, is found to have inoperable carcinoma of the stomach; laparotomy is not performed. He is anorexic, cachectic and very frightened. Give an account of the total responsibilities of the nurse to this patient and his relatives.

4. A mother, aged 40 years, is admitted to your ward in a drowsy state, following a subarachnoid haemorrhage. (a) Describe in detail the observations which should be made and the care which may be given to this patient during the first 48 hours. (b) What investigations may be carried out? (c) Describe the blood supply to the brain.

Section B

5. Describe the total nursing care and management of a patient immediately following tonsillectomy and up to the time of discharge from hospital.

6. (a) Discuss the factors which contribute to the maintenance of a normal blood sugar. (b) Explain why ketones may be present in the urine of a patient with untreated diabetes mellitus. (c) A young patient, admitted to hospital in an unconscious state, is found to have diabetes mellitus. Outline his treatment, medical and nursing, during the 24 hours following admission.

7. (a) Why is it important that the family should be included in the total care of a patient? (b) Discuss the value of unrestricted visiting for patients of all ages and the ways in which the consequent difficulties may be overcome.

8. Discuss the significance of the following and outline the investigations and/or treatment that may ensue in each case: (a) escape of cerebrospinal fluid from the ear of a patient admitted with a head injury; (b) profuse vomiting in a patient who has had a laparotomy; (c) retention of urine in a patient with a spinal lesion; (d) tetany in a patient who has had a subtotal thyroidectomy.

Questions set at the Final State Examination for the Part of the Register for Sick Children's Nurses

February 1976

All Aspects of Nursing Care and Treatment of Sick Children

(Morning)

1. A 9-month-old infant, who weighs 11·0 kg (24 lb 4 oz) is admitted with bronchiolitis. (a) With reference to anatomy and physiology describe the appearance of this infant. (b) Give a detailed account of his nursing care and treatment.

2. (a) Draw a labelled diagram to show the structure of the skin and list its functions. (b) Give a detailed account of the nursing care and treatment for 72 hours following the admission of a 4-year-old girl with either: (i) severe eczema; or (ii) scalds of neck and chest.

3. A 12-year-old girl with a cerebral tumour, who is aware of her prognosis, is admitted for terminal care. (a) Describe the total nursing care required. (b) Discuss the advantages and disadvantages of visitors for this patient.

4. You are in charge of the ward. Give an account of the actions that need to be taken in the following situations: (a) a boy aged 7 years, recently diagnosed as having diabetes mellitus, is missing; (b) a 2-year-old girl bites another child breaking the skin surface; (c) an error in the administration of oral digoxin to an infant has been made.

5. A premature infant who weighs 1·5 kg (3 lb 5 oz) develops either: (a) respiratory distress syndrome; or (b) physiological jaundice (hyperbilirubinaemia). (i) Describe the condition you have chosen. (ii) Give an account of the total nursing care and medical treatment of this infant.

6. An 18-month-old boy has been in the ward for two weeks on gallows traction for a fractured femur. He develops diarrhoea and vomiting. (a) Give an account of the measures that need to be taken to control the spread of infection. (b) Describe the total nursing care of the child including the re-establishment of a normal diet.

7. John is a rather aggressive 4-year-old child, who has Down's syndrome (mongolism). His mother has a new baby and the family live in a high-rise flat. (a) Write short notes on Down's syndrome. (b) Discuss the problems which may arise and the facilities available to assist this family.

(Afternoon)

1. A newborn baby boy weighing 3·4 kg (7 lb 8 oz) is admitted to the ward. He has an intestinal obstruction due to Hirschsprung's disease and requires a colostomy. (a) What is Hirschsprung's disease? (b) List his preoperative care. (c) Describe his postoperative nursing care and management until his discharge home.

2. A 10-year-old boy is admitted to the ward with suspected osteomyelitis of his right tibia. He is acutely ill. (a) List the possible signs and symptoms. (b) Describe how nursing care and medical treatment is given to alleviate these signs and symptoms and to aid recovery.

3. (a) What would make you suspect that a child has sustained non-accidental injuries? A 10-month-old baby girl is admitted to the ward. She is fretful and small for her age. There is evidence of child abuse. (b) Describe how the nursing staff can help this baby during her stay in hospital. (c) Discuss how her preparation for discharge from hospital may be planned and implemented.

4. A 4-year-old girl has ureteric reflux. She is admitted to the ward for reimplantation of both ureters. (a) Explain why this operation may be necessary. (b) Describe the nursing care of this child from the time of operation until her discharge home.

5. How would you help a junior nurse carry out three of the following pro-

cedures: (a) the administration of an intramuscular injection to a 4-year-old child; (b) nasopharyngeal suction prior to feeding a 6-month-old baby; (c) instillation of eye drops to a 3-year-old child; (d) removal of an intravenous infusion from a 6-year-old child?

6. Discuss the advantages and disadvantages from the mother's point of view of being resident in hospital with her child. Relate your answer to the following situations: (a) a baby admitted to hospital for investigations soon after birth; (b) a 5-year-old child who is seriously ill.

7. Choose any one child or infant you have nursed who has undergone cardiac surgery. (a) Describe, with the aid of a diagram, the cardiac lesion. (b) State the age of the patient and the operation which was performed. Describe in detail the nursing care of this patient for the first 48 hours following surgery.

Appendix IV

Questions set at the Examination for the Diploma in Paediatric Nursing of the South African Nursing Council

(Reproduced by permission of the South African Nursing Council)

February 1970

1. A child, 10 years old, is admitted in a coma, presumably diabetic. How would you prove that? Give the nursing care of this patient. What instructions would you give the patient and the mother?

2. Give the cause of convulsions in children. How would you care for a patient having a fit in your ward? Give your report to the doctor in charge.

3. Name the causes of intestinal obstruction in an infant. Give the nursing care of a baby with hypertrophic pyloric stenosis (a) under medical treatment and (b) having had surgical correction.

4. Give the causes of croup (stridor) in infants and young children. Describe the nursing care of patients suffering from the various conditions mentioned.

February 1971

1. (a) Make a list of the nutritional diseases found in children in South Africa. (b) Outline the treatment and nursing care of a 2-year-old child suffering from protein-calorie malnutrition.

2. (a) Discuss the causes of acute diarrhoea in preschool children. (b) Briefly describe the complication which may arise during the disease.

3. What are the complications of: (a) long-term corticosteroid therapy; (b) streptomycin therapy; (c) digoxin therapy; (d) aspirin therapy?

4. Give the signs and symptoms of acute nephritis. Outline the treatment and nursing care of a patient suffering from this disease.

5. Describe the symptoms and signs of congenital pyloric stenosis. Outline the pre- and postoperative care of a baby with pyloric stenosis.

July 1971

1. A 6-year-old child is admitted with 15 per cent burns involving the right hand and arm, face and part of the anterior chest wall. Discuss the treatment and nursing care for the first week.

2. Describe the signs and symptoms of acute pneumonia in a 6-month-old baby and outline the nursing care of the child in the hospital.

3. Describe briefly the physical developmental stages in a normal child up to the age of 6 years.

4. (a) What are the habit-forming drugs and why are they controlled by law? (b) What precautions should a nurse take in the care and administration of these drugs in a ward?

February 1972

1. Outline the clinical features of intestinal obstruction in the newborn. Discuss the preoperative and postoperative nursing care of a baby with oesophageal atresia.

2. An 11-year-old child is admitted fully conscious to the ward with a terminal disease. Discuss the nursing role in this situation under the following headings: (a) The management of the child in the last few days of life; (b) The management of the anxiety and sorrow within the child's family; (c) Helping the other children in the ward over this period; (d) The use of other members of the child's home environment.

3. Write short notes on the dangers of the following procedures and treatment: (a) lumbar puncture; (b) renal biopsy; (c) restraining and not restraining children in hospital; (d) antibiotic therapy.

4. Discuss the signs and symptoms of acute leukaemia in childhood. What diagnostic investigations will be done? Outline the broad principles of treatment and the dangers thereof.

5. What steps would you, as a ward sister, take to prevent cross-infection of gastroenteritis in your ward?

July 1972

1. A 3-month-old baby is admitted to the ward with a harelip and cleft palate for repair of the harelip only. Discuss the pre- and postoperative nursing care of this child.

2. Describe the signs and symptoms of congenital pyloric stenosis. Outline the pre- and postoperative nursing care of a baby with pyloric stenosis.

3. How would you recognise a child suffering from kwashiorkor? Describe the nursing care of a child suffering from this condition and what advice you would give the parents to avoid a recurrence of the disease.

4. What are the basic daily nutritional requirements for a 1-week-old baby weighing 8 lb? How would you artificially feed this baby for the first month of life?

5. Describe in detail an immunisation programme which you would recommend for a child in the first six years of life. Name one contraindication to one of these procedures.

6. Make a list of the major and minor signs and symptoms of rheumatic fever. Describe the nursing care of a 12-year-old child with acute rheumatic fever.

7. Write short notes on (a) bed-wetting; (b) the milestones of normal development in the first two years of life; (c) breath-holding attacks.

February 1973

1. Describe the clinical presentation of intussusception in a baby of 9 months. Outline the postoperative care of this patient.

2. An intelligent 8-year-old child is admitted to hospital for major cardiac surgery. She is accompanied by her parents. Discuss the *psychological* management of this child and her parents on admission and prior to surgery.

3. Make a list of the signs and symptoms of acute laryngotracheobronchitis with special reference to those signs which might indicate the necessity for tracheostomy. Outline the postoperative nursing care for the first 24 hours of a 6-month-old baby with a tracheostomy.

4. Write short notes on the signs and symptoms and emergency treatment of the following poisonings: (i) aspirin; (ii) iron; (iii) paraffin.

5. What steps would you, as a ward sister, take to prevent the spread of gastroenteritis in your ward?

6. Write short notes on: (i) the eruption of primary teeth in the normal child up to the age of 6 years; (ii) the optimum level of fluoride in drinking water for the

formation of sound teeth; (iii) the ages during which fluoride intake will strengthen tooth formation.

February 1974

1. Tabulate the causes of convulsions in childhood. Describe the management of an epileptic child at home.

2. Write short notes on the following: (a) temper tantrums; (b) breath-holding attacks; (c) nocturnal enuresis.

3. What are the symptoms and signs of acute glomerulonephritis in childhood? Describe the nursing care of a 5-year-old child with this disease.

4. Discuss the ward sister's role in helping to keep hospital costs as low as possible.

5. What advice would you give to a mother regarding prevention of disease in her child for the first two years of life?

6. (a) How does a child develop acute osteomyelitis? (b) Describe the clinical manifestations of this disease. (c) Describe the treatment and nursing care of an 8-year-old child suffering from acute osteomyelitis of the right tibia.

February 1975

1. (a) Make a list of the symptoms and signs of iron-deficiency anaemia and the reason for its frequent occurrence in childhood. (b) List the complications connected with the giving of blood transfusions.

2. An 11-year-old child is admitted fully conscious to the ward with a terminal disease. Discuss the nurse's role in this situation under the following headings: (a) the management of the child in the last few days of life; (b) the management of the anxiety and sorrow in the child's family; (c) the use of other members of the child's home environment.

3. Name the complications of the following: (a) long-term corticosteroid therapy; (b) long-term streptomycin therapy; (c) long-term aspirin therapy.

4. Discuss the role of the ward sister with regard to the maintenance of a satisfactory standard of hygiene in her ward.

5. (a) Define the term congenital diaphragmatic hernia. (b) What symptoms would indicate a severe form of this condition in a newborn infant? (c) What is the immediate duty of the nurse if she suspects this condition?

6. (a) What objective measures are generally used to assess the physical progress of an infant or child? (b) Discuss briefly the value of percentile charts with regard to the judgement of the physical progress of a child. (c) Name the clinical observations which would indicate the diagnosis of kwashiorkor.

Appendix V

A Comprehensive List of Short Objective Questions

It is suggested that the answering of these questions will serve as a useful method of revision.

1. How much protein is there in 100 ml of cow's milk?
2. How many calories are there in 100 ml of breast milk?
3. Name three types of congenital heart disease which are amenable to surgical treatment.
4. Define the term 'kernicterus'.
5. Define the term 'infant mortality rate'.
6. Name three important causes of neonatal death.
7. Mention the most important known causes of a mother going into premature labour.
8. What types of congenital abnormalities may be produced in the foetus of a pregnant woman having had rubella?
9. What is the incubation period of measles?
10. Name two complications of mumps.
11. How much feed should a 1500 g premature infant have when 20 days old?
12. How is bilirubin formed?
13. What is Klumpke's paralysis?
14. What is atropine methonitrate (Eumydrin)?
15. How is atropine methonitrate prescribed and in what dose is it usually given to a 3-week-old infant weighing 3·5 kg?
16. Define the term 'stillbirth rate'.
17. How much vitamin C should a low birth weight infant, 4 weeks of age, receive?
18. How is milk pasteurised and why?
19. What diseases may be transmitted by cow's milk?
20. In what form is the carbohydrate present in breast milk?
21. What should be the circumference of the head of a normal infant at 6 months of age?
22. How much should a normal boy of 5 years weigh?
23. What is the average length of a 34-week preterm infant?
24. What amount of fat is present in a litre of cow's milk?
25. Define the term 'supplementary feed'.
26. Which antibiotic may cause staining of the teeth?
27. How does a heterozygous Rh-positive father differ from one who is homozygous Rh positive?
28. Name three causes of constipation in an infant.
29. What is the incubation period of viral hepatitis type B?
30. Name three causes of stomatitis.
31. Name the parasite causing threadworm infestation.
32. Name a drug (anthelmintic) useful in the treatment of roundworm infestation.
33. What organism causes amoebic dysentery?
34. Name the nasal accessory sinuses.
35. Which antibiotics are indicated for the treatment of brucellosis?

36. What are the two commonest cyanotic congenital heart diseases?
37. Name three drugs used in the treatment of tuberculosis.
38. What is the commonest type of anaemia found in childhood?
39. What is Hutchinson's triad of symptoms and in what disease is this triad found?
40. Name three causes of rectal bleeding in childhood.
41. What is a cephalhaematoma?
42. What causes thrush?
43. Name three causes of stridor.
44. Name two possible causes of cerebral palsy.
45. Which parts of the body may be affected by ringworm?
46. What is a tic?
47. Which antibiotic may cause jaundice in the newborn?
48. Define a choreiform movement.
49. How does a choreiform movement differ from an athetoid one?
50. What causes scabies and what is the best application to apply for the treatment of this disease?
51. What causes erythema nodosum?
52. Mention four causes of steatorrhoea in a child.
53. Name two indications for tonsillectomy.
54. What is Still's disease?
55. What is the risk of carditis complicating an attack of Sydenham's chorea?
56. Define the term 'neonatal mortality rate'.
57. What is a complementary feed?
58. What is 'three month colic'?
59. Mention four dangers to which a low birth weight infant is liable.
60. What is the commonest type of skull fracture seen in a newborn infant?
61. How much vitamin K_1 should you give as a prophylactic dose in a newborn low birth weight infant of 1500 g?
62. Define the term 'marasmus'.
63. What causes nits?
64. What is the incubation period of scarlet fever?
65. Name two serious complications of diphtheria.
66. What is pica?
67. How does phenobarbitone affect jaundice of the newborn and what is the mechanism?
68. How many kilocalories does a 4·5 kg infant require?
69. How much calcium is there in a litre of cow's milk?
70. Define the term 'low birth weight infant'.
71. What causes scarlet fever?
72. By what age should the anterior fontanelle close?
73. Name two diseases which may be associated with late closure of the anterior fontanelle.
74. How tall should a child of 5 years be?
75. At what stage of pregnancy may German measles (rubella) endanger the foetus?
76. What is perinatal mortality?
77. Name a disease which may produce blindness in a low birth weight infant and what may cause it.
78. What is the commonest organism causing neonatal meningitis?
79. Why is vitamin C given to low birth weight infants?
80. How is cystic fibrosis (fibrocystic disease of the pancreas) transmitted as a hereditary disease?
81. Which sex does Sydenham's chorea usually affect?
82. Which heart valve does rheumatic carditis affect most commonly?
83. Name one clinical sign of nutritional rickets.

84. What is the normal daily requirement of vitamin D in infancy?
85. In what way may diabetes mellitus present clinically in a child?
86. Name two conditions in which an infant may have snuffles.
87. What fluid is used to perform a stomach washout in congenital hypertrophic pyloric stenosis?
88. In what condition is desferrioxamine (Desferal) used?
89. Name the type of tapeworm caused by 'measly' pork.
90. Name two anthelmintics for the treatment of taeniasis (tapeworm infestation).
91. What symptoms can giardia infestation cause in a child?
92. What is the incubation period of typhoid fever?
93. Name two causes of vomiting in an infant aged 16 days.
94. What is the cause of verrucae?
95. Name two diseases transmitted as a sex-linked condition.
96. How much carbohydrate is there present in cow's milk?
97. What is the Eustachian tube?
98. What is the commonest cause of jaundice in a child of school-going age?
99. At what age do the deciduous canine teeth erupt?
100. Name two congenital abnormalities found more often in females.
101. Name the immunoglobulins.
102. Name two conditions where human immunoglobulin may be administered.
103. Name three causes of epistaxis.
104. What investigation may be done to confirm the diagnosis of cystic fibrosis?
105. Name a drug used in the treatment of a giardia infection of the bowel.
106. Smallpox vaccination. Name three complications which may follow this procedure.
107. What part does factor VIII play in the blood-clotting mechanism?
108. Name two good reasons why breast feeding is superior to artificial feeding.
109. Name two causes for short stature.
110. What is the Guthrie test?

INDEX